A Parent's Guide to Medical Emergencies

FIRST AID FOR YOUR CHILD

Janet Zand, OMD
Rachel Walton, RN
Bob Rountree, MD

D0187503

Avery Publishing Group
Garden City Park, New York

The medical information and procedures contained in this book are based upon the careful research and professional experiences of the authors. The recommended procedures should be followed until professional help can take over. Taking a certified first aid course that includes life-saving emergency procedures is suggested for any person who cares for a child on a regular basis. This book is as timely and accurate as its publisher and authors can make it; nevertheless, they disclaim all liablity and cannot be held responsible for any problems that may arise from its use.

Cover Designer: William Gonzalez
Text Illustrator: John Wincek
Typesetter: Al Berotti
In-House Editor: Marie Caratozzolo
Printer: Paragon Press, Honesdale, PA

Avery Publishing Group
120 Old Broadway
Garden City Park, NY 11040
1–800–548–5757

Library of Congress Cataloging-in-Publication Data

Zand, Janet.
    A parent's guide to medical emergencies : first aid for your child
/ by Janet Zand, Rachel Walton, Bob Rountree.
        p. cm.
    Includes index.
    ISBN 0–89529–736–1
    1. Pediatric emergencies—Popular works. 2. First aid in illness
and injury. I. Walton, Rachel. II. Rountree, Bob. III. Title.
RJ370.Z36 1997
618.92'0252—dc21   97–7955
                                                            CIP

Copyright © 1997 by Janet Zand

All rights reserved. No part of this publication may be reproduced, stored in a retrieval system, or transmitted, in any form or by any means, electronic, photocopying, recording, or otherwise, without the prior written permission of the copyright owner.

10 9 8 7 6 5 4 3 2 1

Quick Emergency Reference Guide

Contents

■ PART THREE   *The Emergencies*

Preface

Our desire in writing this book is to provide parents a holistic context within which to handle a medical emergency. Our greatest hope is that no parent will ever have to endure the challenge of seeing their child badly hurt. Modern medicine offers us great knowledge and skill in treating a serious physical crisis. Natural medicine offers therapeutics that will help strengthen and balance a child following a medical emergency. It is necessary to support the body and restore it to full health. Most importantly, remember the heart and spirit by doing what you do best—paying close attention to your child through listening and loving. Honor what you know to be true; respect your unique capabilities as a parent.

To this end, we thank Rudy Shur for his continued support, Marie Caratozzolo for her skillful editing, and Peter Levine, Ph.D. for his significant contribution to the work of healing stress and trauma in the body. We also thank the teachers, colleagues, parents, children, family, and friends who warm our hearts and keep us on track.

Part One

Safety Measures

Introduction

No matter how careful a parent you are, you cannot prevent all of the medical emergencies that can arise as your children grow up. The best way to avoid a medical emergency is through precautionary measures. Yet, even the most safety-conscious parents can find their children facing one medical emergency or another. A responsible parent must be prepared to handle such crises.

Part One begins with a section on *Home Safety*. As accidents are the leading cause of injury and death among young children, childproofing your home against such mishaps is a wise move. Safety checklists are provided for every area in and around the home.

The section on *Emergency Preparedness* beginning on page 12, suggests important steps for you to take, such as posting emergency telephone numbers and teaching your child how to use the telephone to summon help, in order to act quickly and effectively in a crisis situation.

The final section of Part One is *Understanding Childhood Trauma After an Emergency*. A frightening episode (even one that may not seem frightening to you as an adult) can have a psychologically negative impact on your child. Information provided in this section is designed to help you recognize the signs that may indicate your child has been traumatized. Also presented are techniques that you can employ to help your child deal with and eventually resolve the trauma.

Home Safety

Accidents are the leading cause of injury and death among children ages one to fourteen years. It makes sense to do everything you can to childproof your home and surroundings against accidents.

Your child's age and developmental level will determine the kinds of hazards he is likely to encounter. Infants are attracted to bright and shiny objects. They are curious about everything, and everything they touch goes into their mouths, creating a risk of choking or poisoning. As a baby learns to roll over, sit, crawl, and reach, he can tumble off a bed or changing table, pull a piece of filmy plastic over his face, or slip under water in the bathtub.

Toddlers also are extremely curious. They are attracted to bright packaging, and are learning to open things. Often, they succeed. They are learning to walk and will venture out of sight from time to time. Because the "terrible twos" are a time when little ones typically start to assert their independence by saying "no," it can be difficult to enforce limits. Toddlers especially are at risk for poisoning, choking, and getting burned.

Older children are mastering new skills, such as biking and swimming. They are likely to be off exploring in secret places with friends, heedless of dangers. Bicycle accidents, near-drownings, poisoning from berries and outdoor plants, and getting lost are among the potential hazards for this age group. Most authorities recommend gentle but persistent warnings against accepting gifts or other enticements from strangers, as young children tend to be trusting of anyone who acts nice to them.

Teenagers typically feel invincible and immortal. In their desire for independence, they often push parents to the limit. Often, teenagers are under intense peer pressure to experiment with dangerous substances, to flirt with danger, to dare anything. This age group is at risk for car accidents, bicycle and motorcycle accidents, sports injuries, and toxic ingestion of drugs and alcohol.

Children of any age who are hyperactive, visually or hearing impaired, or physically or mentally handicapped tend to suffer more accidents than other children do. In addition, some children are simply more curious and more adventuresome than others. Some constantly rebel against authority of any kind and continually test their parents' resolve. Such children can be exhausting, but it is your responsibility as a parent to persevere. Remember that children need appropriate limits; without them, a child will feel lost and insecure, even unloved.

Talk to your child. Using language and explanations your child understands, teach safety considerations both inside and outside the home. It's much more effective to explain to your child how he could get hurt in a given circumstance than it is to say crossly, "Don't do it because I say so."

Be especially patient with a very young child. Young children have short attention spans and may not have the ability to rationalize and retain information. A young child may be unable to follow directions or understand the consequences of certain actions. Repetition is effective. Even if you have to go over a problem again and again, keep at it until your child understands.

Keep in mind also that children are natural mimics; they imitate the adults around them. It's up to you to set a safe example. As you teach your child to fasten his seat belt, you must also fasten yours. Obey street crossing signals. Don't walk your child across a street against the light. Don't drink and drive.

Try to scan your home carefully with the curious eyes of a child. Get down on your hands and knees and crawl around. Notice that the electrical sockets are at a crawling child's eye level, easily within reach and tempting to poke at. Look for bright, shiny objects, items a child might pop into his mouth. Spot the things your child might grab or pull on with disastrous results. For example, tugging on the trailing edge of a table cover or the loop of an electrical cord could bring a tableful of dishes or a heavy lamp crashing to the floor. At a child's eye level, you'll be able to spot potential hazards more easily.

Be prepared. Not all accidents can be prevented, so knowing how to handle emergencies is an important safety precaution. Learn cardiopulmonary resuscitation (CPR) and first aid. The Red Cross offers courses in first aid, as do many hospitals. The important thing is to learn these procedures before you need to use them. Make sure any course you take includes a thorough grounding in infant and child CPR, and take a refresher course every year.

Assemble and keep, in a convenient but secure location, a home health kit stocked with the basics for dealing with illness and injury (see page 15). Check expiration dates periodically and replace any outdated products promptly.

Safety Checklist

The safety checklist that follows will help you limit injuries and child-proof your home.

THROUGHOUT YOUR HOME

☐ Make sure that every room in your home has a working smoke and carbon monoxide detector. If detectors are wired in, it's a good idea to have a battery-operated backup in case of loss of electricity. Check and replace batteries as required.

☐ Close off electrical outlets with safety devices. These are available in most hardware stores.

☐ Keep floors clean of pins, buttons, food, and any other small objects a child could pick up and put in his mouth.

☐ Put colorful stickers on picture windows and glass doors at your child's eye level, so that he can see them and will not accidentally run into them.

☐ Remove heavy or sharp objects, such as picture frames, vases, and lamps, from tables, or move them away from the edges so that your child cannot pull them over.

☐ Remove tablecloths that might be grabbed and pulled off.

☐ Keep securely closed safety gates at the tops and bottoms of stairs.

☐ Secure windows so that your child cannot reach an open window and fall out. Open windows from the top; keep screens secure. Do not put furniture in front of a window; this offers a path up to the sill.

☐ Tie dangling curtain, drapery, and blind cords out of reach, especially those located near a crib or bed. Children can become entangled in such cords and suffocate.

☐ Keep plastic bags, which can cause suffocation, out of reach of your child at all times.

☐ Use only nontoxic and lead-free paints in your home.

☐ Keep all cleaning products, paints, gardening and hobby supplies, and any other dangerous substances out of reach of your child in a locked cabinet.

☐ Keep all fireplaces securely screened and free of ashes and soot, which can be inhaled by a curious child.

☐ If any work is being done in your home, talk to the workers about safety considerations for your child. Keep them aware of your child and your safety concerns. Ask them about special child hazards that might be involved in their work. Keep dirty drop cloths away from your child's sleeping and playing areas; be sure tools are properly stored, out of reach, at the end of the work day; keep lids on cans of paints, varnishes, solvents, and other products at all times; and create a safe place for your child, away from dust, nails, tools, splinters, paints, and fumes.

☐ When using any potentially harmful item, such as a cleaning product, do not let it out of your sight. If you need to leave a room to answer the door or the phone, take the product with you.

☐ Call your local Poison Control Center for information on preventing poisoning (*see* listings beginning on page 155). Most centers will send you free literature with detailed instructions on how to poison-proof your home, as well as on what to do (and what *not* to do) in case of poisoning. "Mr. Yuk" stickers can be obtained from the Poison Control Center. Place them on potentially poisonous materials. Keep in mind that vitamins with iron are a common cause of poisoning.

☐ All children are fascinated by fire and may eventually want to experiment with matches. Keep matches well hidden and securely out of reach.

☐ Set the temperature for the hot water heater in your home no higher than 120°F. It takes only five seconds for 140°F water to cause a severe third-degree burn, but it takes a full three minutes to get a third-degree burn from 120°F water. Those extra minutes may provide enough time for you to snatch your child out of harm's way and prevent a nasty scald.

MEALTIMES

- ☐ Do not let an infant or young child eat alone. Always keep a watchful eye out to prevent choking.
- ☐ Eat slowly and chew food thoroughly, and teach your child to do the same. Sit down to eat. Make mealtime a relaxed, happy time.
- ☐ Cut food into small, bite-sized pieces for your child. Teach him to take small bites from crackers or cookies.
- ☐ Do not give a young child hot dogs, nuts, raisins, popcorn, or other similar foods. Young children may not chew finger foods sufficiently to prevent choking.
- ☐ Don't permit your toddler to eat while he is engaged in play activity. It's too easy for a bite to go down wrong if he takes a tumble.

IN THE KITCHEN

- ☐ Keep all knives and other sharp objects out of reach.
- ☐ Never store any potentially harmful object in food jars or food storage containers.
- ☐ When cooking, use the back burners whenever possible, and be sure to keep pot handles turned toward the stove so that your child cannot reach or bump a hot pot.
- ☐ Keep appliances, such as the toaster, food processor, and blender, unplugged and well away from counter edges.
- ☐ Cover the garbage disposal.
- ☐ Place secure plastic fasteners (available in most hardware stores) on cabinet doors to keep your child out of cupboards that hold glass, china, cleaning products, and other potentially harmful substances.
- ☐ Keep a fire extinguisher in a handy location near the stove, but make sure it is out of your child's reach.

IN THE BATHROOM

- ☐ Apply nonslip surfaces to the bottom of the bathtub.
- ☐ *Never* leave an infant or young child in the bathtub alone. If you must leave the room to answer the phone or door, wrap your little one in a towel and take him with you.

☐ Keep all medicines and supplements out of reach. Throw away old medicines and prescriptions.

☐ Do not leave medicines or cleaning products on a counter within reach of your child.

☐ If you store potentially harmful products in a cupboard under your bathroom sink, secure the cabinet with a plastic fastener.

☐ Do not leave a razor within your child's reach.

☐ Keep the toilet lid down.

IN YOUR CHILD'S PLAY AREA

☐ Do not give your infant toys that are small enough to fit into his mouth.

☐ Do not give your child any toy that has small parts that could break off.

☐ A teething infant should never be permitted to play with a toy that is filled with liquid or gel.

☐ Check your child's playthings regularly for breakage and keep them in good repair. If repainting is necessary, use only nontoxic and lead-free paints.

☐ Choose age-appropriate toys carefully. Follow the age guidelines on the packaging. Be aware that these guidelines refer primarily to the ages a child must be to use a toy safely. Thus, if a toy is recommended for children ages two through six, it may not be safe for a child under two, even if the child seems old enough for it in other ways. Also keep an eye out for sharp edges, small parts that could loosen (glass eyes, for example), parts that could break, or any electrical wiring that might not be perfect.

☐ Choose toys made from nontoxic materials.

IN THE BEDROOM

☐ If your baby sleeps in a crib, make sure to use one that meets current federal safety standards. It is possible for an infant to be strangled if his head becomes wedged between the bars of a crib.

☐ Protect a sleeping child by making sure he wears flame-retardant clothing.

☐ Never leave your infant alone on a changing table; always keep one hand on your baby. Kicking and wriggling can propel him off the edge.

☐ Keep bureau and table tops clean and clear of sharp objects that could cut your child.

☐ Small objects, such as jewelry and safety pins, can cause choking. Keep them securely out of your child's reach.

REGARDING PETS AND OTHER ANIMALS

☐ Keep a watchful eye as infants interact with pets. Babies can't defend themselves against being scratched or bitten.

☐ Young children should be taught never to approach a strange animal.

☐ Young children should be monitored while playing with family pets. It can take only a moment for play to turn rough.

☐ After playing with pets, children should have their hands washed thoroughly (with special attention to fingernails) to help prevent the possible spread of germs and/or parasites.

☐ Make sure your child does not come in contact with animal feces, which may be contaminated. Designate a separate fenced outdoor area as your dog's toilet facility. "Scoop" the area regularly to keep it clean so that he doesn't bring any fecal matter into the house on his feet. For cats, put the litter box in a place that is inaccessible to your child. Keep the litter box scrupulously clean.

☐ Make sure your pets get good routine health care, including regular worming and flea treatment. Keep your child away from any animal that is obviously ill, and take sick pets to the veterinarian promptly for treatment.

OTHER AREAS

☐ Prevent cuts and choking by making sure your sewing area is clean and clear of buttons, pins, needles, and scissors. Such objects are enticing to children.

☐ Keep your sewing machine unplugged when not in use, and the cord securely out of reach.

☐ Garages, tool sheds, and workshops should be securely locked and off-limits to young children.

OUTSIDE YOUR HOME

☐ When your child is a passenger in an automobile, keep him securely buckled in an appropriate safety restraint at all times. Consumer magazines, the United States Department of Transportation, and the National Child Passenger Safety Association (located in Ardmore, Pennsylvania) can provide information on approved child restraint systems.

☐ Teach your child to cross streets safely. Young children should be taught to cross a street only in the company of an adult, never alone.

☐ Make sure your child wears appropriate protective gear when engaging in sports activities. A helmet should be worn for bicycling, horseback riding, skiing, skateboarding, and roller blading, as well as organized sports like baseball, football, hockey, and lacrosse. Eye protection is recommended for children who play baseball, hockey, racquet sports, football, basketball, and golf. Goggles are useful for protecting eyes from chlorine and other chemicals while swimming. Other types of protective gear that may be appropriate include knee pads, elbow pads, shin guards, mouth guards, and padded gloves.

☐ Teach children to swim and teach them water safety.

☐ Never leave a child alone near a swimming pool, lake, pond, or any other body of water. There are many instances of drowning and near-drowning that occur because young children are left unsupervised. Swimming pools should be securely fenced.

☐ When your child is riding in a boat, make sure he is wearing a life jacket.

☐ Before allowing your child to skate on a frozen pond, check with local authorities to make sure the ice is safe.

☐ Keep your child's playground equipment in good repair. Put a cushioning layer of sand under slides, swings, and jungle gyms to soften a possible fall.

☐ Always supervise a young child when he is playing outside. Be sure to keep him well away from the street. Teach your child never to chase a ball, another child, or a pet into the street.

☐ Do not grow poisonous plants either inside or outside your home. The ivy and the split-leaf philodendron that look so pretty on your end tables, as well as the flowering azaleas and daffodils that brighten your yard, can be lethal if ingested. Some common plants that should be avoided are apricot, azalea, Boston ivy, caladium, castor bean, chokeberry, daffodil (jonquil, narcissus), dumb cane (dieffenbachia), emerald duke, English ivy, foxglove, hen and chicks (lantana), hydrangea, jimsonweed, lily of the valley, mistletoe, morning glory, nightshade, oleander, parlor ivy (philodendron), poison ivy, poison oak, poison sumac, rhododendron, rhubarb, split-leaf philodendron, sweet pea, tulip, and wisteria.

☐ Children should never be permitted to play with fireworks. Most states prohibit the sale of fireworks to individuals, but people still manage to obtain them. Every year, some children suffer severe burns — or worse — from accidents connected with fireworks.

☐ Insist that your teenager take a driver's education course before getting his driver's license. This shouldn't be difficult; most high schools provide driving instruction. "Driver's Ed" classes are an eagerly anticipated milestone for most teenagers.

☐ Never drink and drive. Teach your teenager about the consequences and very real dangers of drinking and driving, or accepting a ride from anyone who has been drinking.

Not all accidents are preventable, of course, but many are. Thinking ahead is the key. Stay one step ahead of your child. By childproofing the areas in and around your home, you can protect against many home accidents, and also keep to a minimum the hazards your child will encounter outside.

Emergency Preparedness

No matter how careful and loving a parent you are, you cannot prevent all of the accidents and emergencies that can arise while your children are growing up. But you can take measures so that you will be prepared to act quickly and effectively should an emergency arise.

EMERGENCY TELEPHONE NUMBERS

Post emergency telephone numbers near every telephone in your home. This can save precious time in any emergency, for you or for anyone else who is caring for your child. We urge you to take this precaution now, while you are thinking about it. If there is no 911 emergency service in your area, these numbers should include that of your local hospital for ambulance/paramedic service. Also post numbers for your local fire department, Poison Control Center (*see* listings beginning on page 155), police department, and your child's doctor and dentist. It is also helpful to post the numbers of a neighbor, friend, or family member who can help in a crisis situation.

If your telephone is the type that allows you to program numbers for automatic dialing, enter these emergency numbers into the phone as well, and label the appropriate keys clearly. Some telephone models come with keys already labeled for police, fire, and other emergency numbers, which makes this even easier. However, you should not consider this a substitute for keeping emergency numbers on hand in written form. It is possible for programmed numbers to be erased accidentally, so you should still keep a list of emergency telephone numbers in a convenient location.

When your child is old enough to understand, teach her to respond to emergencies. Children as young as three years old have been known

12

to use the telephone to summon emergency help. Teach your child how to dial 911 for emergency assistance if this service is available in your area (or, if not, how to dial 0 for operator), and have your child practice this skill. Use a toy telephone or simply hold the disconnect button down on your regular phone and practice with your child so that she becomes accustomed to the procedure. Help your child understand the appropriate use of this number. Also, make sure your child can recite her full name, address, and telephone number.

DESIGNATED SURROGATES

Choose and empower surrogates who can act in your stead if an emergency arises when you cannot be reached, and include their telephone numbers in the emergency list. Designate adults you trust, perhaps your child's grandparents, perhaps good friends, to make decisions in any emergency involving your child. If you have established a close and caring relationship with your child's health care provider, you might wish to empower him or her to make any necessary medical decisions involving your child. Give your surrogates written permission to act for you, such as a limited power of attorney. Your surrogates should keep this important document where it can be found easily if they must respond to an emergency, and you should give copies to your child's physician. Should an occasion ever arise when you cannot be reached immediately, your designated surrogates will be able to act. Written permission from a parent or designated guardian is sometimes required before certain life-saving measures can be taken.

MEDIC ALERT

If you have a child with a special medical problem, obtain a Medic Alert bracelet to ensure that he will receive the right care if something happens away from home. If your child is allergic to penicillin or other medication, sulfites, or bee stings, for example, it will enable him to receive prompt and appropriate treatment for an allergic reaction. Without a Medic Alert bracelet, a teenager with diabetes who is suffering from the typical symptoms of low blood sugar could be misdiagnosed as being intoxicated and fail to receive necessary treatment. Medic Alert information is especially important for a young child who may not be able to communicate well, or for any child who has a disorder that can cause loss of consciousness.

Without Medic Alert information, health care personnel could be working in the dark and wasting precious time. Medic Alert is the only emergency medical identification service endorsed by the American College of Emergency Physicians, the American Hospital Association, and every national pharmacy association. For more information, call Medic Alert at 800–432–5378.

FIRST AID TRAINING

Primary child care providers in every household should take a good course in emergency first aid that includes infant and childhood cardiopulmonary resuscitation (CPR) procedures and first aid for choking. We hope that you will never be called upon to use these skills, but there is simply no substitute for the hands-on training and practice in these lifesaving techniques that such a course provides. See important lifesaving techniques and procedures in Part Two.

THE WELL-STOCKED HOME HEALTH KIT

Every home should have a well-stocked home health kit. A good kit includes not only the bare essentials for dealing with emergencies, but also basic medicines that are used over and over again for common illnesses (*see* Assembling a Home Health Kit on page 15).

Every health kit should include such basic items as an ace bandage, a sling, a hot water bottle, an ice bag, adhesive bandages, sterile gauze pads, and adhesive tape. Tweezers, scissors, sterilized needles, and a thermometer are other basic necessities. Rubbing alcohol, hydrogen peroxide, or another disinfectant is needed for cleaning wounds and sterilizing needles and tweezers. If your child is allergic to insect bites or stings, a prescription inset-bite kit that contains adrenaline (such as Ana-Guard) is another essential item. Finally, every home health kit should include syrup of ipecac. Used to induce vomiting, *syrup of ipecac is to be taken only at the direction of a doctor or Poison Control Center.* (For information on administering syrup of ipecac, *see* page 153).

In addition to the bare essentials, there are a number of conventional over-the-counter medicines that should be kept on hand for common illnesses. These include acetaminophen (such as children's Tylenol or Tempra) or ibuprofen (such as children's Advil, Nuprin, or Pediaprofen), an antihistamine (such as Benadryl or Chlor-Trimeton), and an antiseptic ointment (such as bacitracin or Betadine). A decongestant (such as Sudafed) is also essential.

Assembling a Home Health Kit

Assembling a home health kit will give you a good base for treating the most common childhood illnesses and injuries. Begin putting it together now, so that if your child does get hurt or sick, the right treatments and remedies will be close at hand. Use the checklist that follows as a guide to some of the most important elements for a variety of different treatment approaches.

Bare Essentials

- Ace bandage.
- Adhesive bandages (Band-Aids).
- Bulb syringe.
- Hot water bottle.
- Ice bag.
- Prescription insect bite kit containing adrenaline (such as Ana-Guard) if your child is allergic to bites or stings.

- Rubbing alcohol, hydrogen peroxide, or witch hazel, for disinfecting wounds and sterilizing needles and tweezers.
- Scissors with rounded tips.
- Sling and safety pins.
- Sterile gauze pads and adhesive tape.

- SAM splint.*
- Sterile razor blade.
- Sterilized needle.
- Syrup of ipecac. *Caution:* Syrup of ipecac should not be used except at the direction of a doctor or Poison Control Center.
- Thermometer.
- Tweezers.

Conventional Medicines

- Acetaminophen (such as Tylenol, Tempra, or the equivalent) or ibuprofen (Advil, Nuprin, Pedia-Profen, and others).

- An antihistamine (such as Benadryl or Chlor-Trimeton).
- An antiseptic ointment (such as bacitracin or Betadine).

- A decongestant (such as Sudafed).
- Emetrol syrup.
- Milk of Magnesia.
- Pepto-Bismol.

Herbal Medicines

- Aloe vera gel.
- Calendula ointment or gel.

- Echinacea tincture.
- Goldenseal tincture.
- Gotu kola.

- Peppermint tea.
- Traumeel ointment.
- Chamomile tea.

* An emergency splint made of foam-lined laminated aluminum.

Homeopathic Remedies

- *Aconite.*
- *Apis.*
- *Arnica.*
- *Arsenicum.*

- *Belladonna.*
- *Ferrum phosphoricum.*
- *Hypericum.*

- *Ledum.*
- *Rhus tox.*
- *Urtica urens.*

Flower Essences

- Aspen.

- Bach Flower Rescue Remedy.

- Mimulus.

Miscellaneous

- Apple or grape juice, or applesauce, to mix with herbs or crushed tablets.

- Eyedropper or needleless syringe to administer liquid medicines.
- Smelling salts.

- Honey, barley malt, or rice bran syrup.
- Save•A•Tooth solution (*see* page 173).

Certain therapeutics—herbals, homeopathics, and flower remedies—are important in helping the body to heal and to further stabilize once an emergency has passed. Essential herbal medicines to be included in your home health kit are aloe vera gel, calendula ointment or gel, chamomile tea, echinacea tincture, goldenseal tincture, gotu kola, peppermint tea, and traumeel ointment. Basic homeopathic remedies include *Aconite, Apis, Arnica, Arsenicum, Belladonna, Ferrum phosphoricum, Hypericum, Ledum,* and *Rhus tox.* Finally, basic flower essences, such as Bach Flower Rescue Remedy (also called Five Flower Formula and Calming Essence), aspen, and mimulus, should be included in your home health kit.

Wherever appropriate, these natural therapeutics have been suggested under the General Recommendation section of the emergency entries. For further information on these natural remedies, consult a qualified health care professional who is well-versed in their use. You may also refer to the book *Smart Medicine for a Healthier Child* by Janet Zand, Rachel Walton, and Bob Rountree (Garden City Park, NY: Avery Publishing Group, 1994). This A-to-Z reference of common childhood health problems provides detailed information on both natural and conventional treatments for infants and children.

Warning

Your home health kit should be stored in a location that is convenient but securely locked and away from or out of reach of children. Check the kit about every three months or so to replace any products that have been used up or have passed their expiration date.

Before giving any medication to a child, be sure you know what you are treating. Read labels on all medications and carefully follow instructions. For proper dosage amounts for commonly used over-the-counter medications, refer to the chart below. Whenever there is any question regarding the proper use of any medication—prescription or over-the-counter—always consult your doctor or other qualified health care professional before administering.

Proper Dosages for Common Over-the-Counter Medications

Provided below is a listing of the proper dosages for the most commonly used over-the-counter medications for children. Before giving any medication to a child, be sure you know what you are treating. In general, consult your doctor before giving any medication to a child less than two years old.

Weight	Age	Dosage	Cautions
Acetaminophen (Infant's Tylenol, Tempra, St. Joseph's Aspirin-Free) 80 mg/0.8ml = 1 dropperful			
Under 24 pounds	Under 2 years	Consult your doctor.	Do not give to a child with kidney or liver disease.
24–35 pounds	2–3 years	2 dropperfuls (4–6 hours)	
Acetaminophen (Children's Liquid Tylenol, Tempra) 160 mg/5ml = 1 teaspoon			
Under 24 pounds	Under 2 years	Consult your doctor.	Do not give to a child with kidney or liver disease.
24–35 pounds	2–3 years	1 teaspoon (every 4 hours)	
36–47 pounds	4–5 years	1 ½ teaspoons (every 4 hours)	
48–59 pounds	6–8 years	2 teaspoons (every 4 hours)	
60–71 pounds	9–10 years	2 ½ teaspoons (every 4 hours)	
72–95 pounds	11 years	3 teaspoons (every 4 hours)	

Weight	Age	Dosage	Cautions
Acetaminophen (Children's Tylenol Chewable Tablets) 80 mg per tablet			
Under 24 pounds	Under 2 years	Consult your doctor.	Do not give to a child with kidney or liver disease.
24–35 pounds	2–3 years	2 tablets (every 4 hours)	
36–47 pounds	4–5 years	3 tablets (every 4 hours)	
48–59 pounds	6–8 years	4 tablets (every 4 hours)	
60–71 pounds	9–10 years	5 tablets (every 4 hours)	
72–95 pounds	11 years	6 tablets (every 4 hours)	
Aspirin			
Any weight	Under twenty years.	Consult your doctor.	Do not give aspirin unless your doctor specifically recommends it. Aspirin has been associated with the development of Reye's syndrome, a potentially life-threatening disease.
Benadryl (Diphenhydramine Hydrochloride)			
48–95 pounds	6–12 years	12.5–25 mg (4–6 hours)	No more than 150 mg in one day
Over 95 pounds	Over 12 years	25–50 mg (4–6 hours)	No more than 300 mg in one day
Ibuprofen (Children's Advil or Motrin) 100 mg/5 ml = 1 Teaspoon			
Under 24 pounds	Under 2 years	Consult your doctor.	Do not give to a child with kidney or liver disease.
24–35 pounds	2–3 years	1 teaspoon (6–8 hours)	
36–47 pounds	4–5 years	1½ teaspoons (6–8 hours)	
48–59 pounds	6–8 years	2 teaspoons (6–8 hours)	
60–71 pounds	9–10 years	2½ teaspoons (6–8 hours)	
72–95 pounds	11 years	1 tablespoon (6–8 hours)	
Syrup of Ipecac			
	Over 1 year	1 tablespoon followed by 8–16 ounces water. If no vomiting within 20 minutes, repeat dose once more only.	Check with doctor or Poison Control Center (*see* page 155 for listings) before giving ipecac. Depending on substance swallowed, ipecac may or may not be indicated.

Understanding Childhood Trauma After an Emergency

Johnny, age five, proudly riding his first bicycle, hits loose gravel and careens into a tree. He is momentarily knocked unconscious. Getting up amid a flow of tears, he feels disoriented and somehow different. His parents hug him, console him, and put him back on the bike, all the while praising his courage. They do not realize how stunned and frightened he is.

Years after the forgotten incident, John, driving with his wife and children, swerves to avoid an oncoming car. He freezes in the midst of the turn. Fortunately, the other driver is able to maneuver successfully and avoid catastrophe.

One morning, several days later, John begins to feel restless while driving to work. His heart starts racing and pounding; his hands become cold and sweaty. Feeling threatened and trapped, he has a sudden impulse to jump out of the car and run. He realizes the "craziness" of his feelings, and gradually the symptoms subside. A vague and nagging apprehension, however, persists throughout most of the day at work. Returning home that evening without incident, he feels relieved.

The next morning, John leaves early to avoid traffic and stays late, discussing business with some colleagues. When he arrives home, he is irritable and edgy. He argues with his wife and barks at the children. He goes to bed early, yet wakes up covered with sweat in the middle of the night and faintly recalling a dream in which his car is sliding out of control. More fretful nights follow.

DELAYED TRAUMATIC REACTIONS

John is experiencing a delayed reaction to the bike accident he had as a child. Incredible as it may seem, post-traumatic reactions of this type are common. After working for more than twenty years with people suffering from trauma, I can safely say that at least 75 percent of my clients have traumatic symptoms that remained dormant for a significant period of time before surfacing. For most people, the interval between the event and the onset of symptoms is between six and eighteen months; for others, the latency period lasts for years or even decades. In both instances, the reactions are triggered by seemingly insignificant events.

Of course, not every childhood accident produces a delayed traumatic reaction. Some have no residual effect at all. Others, including those viewed as "minor" and forgotten incidents of childhood, can have significant aftereffects. A fall, a seemingly benign operation, the loss of a parent through death or divorce, severe illness (particularly one accompanied by high fever or poisoning), even circumcision and other routine medical procedures can all cause traumatic reactions later in life *depending on how the child experiences them at the time they occur.*

Of these traumatic antecedents, medical procedures are by far the most common and potentially the most impacting. Many clinical proceedings needlessly amplify the fear of an already frightened child. Infants about to undergo some routines, for example, are strapped into "papooses" to keep them from moving. A child struggling so much that he or she needs to be tied down, however, is a child too frightened to be restrained without suffering consequences. Likewise, a child who is severely frightened is not one to be anesthetized, at least not until a sense of tranquillity has been restored. Children can even be traumatized by insensitively administered enemas or thermometers.

Much of the trauma associated with these and other medical procedures could be prevented if healthcare providers encouraged parents to stay with their children, to explain as much as is possible in advance, and to delay interventions until their children are calm. The problem is that too few professionals really understand what trauma is about and what lasting and pervasive effects these procedures can have. Although medical personnel are often concerned, they may need more information—from you, the consumer.

WHAT CAUSES TRAUMA?

At the root of a traumatic reaction is the 280-million-year-old heritage that we share with nearly every crawling creature on earth—a heritage that resides in the area of the nervous system known as the reptilian brain. Primitive responses that originate in this portion of the brain help the organism protect itself against circumstances that are potentially damaging to survival. Animals in the wild routinely encounter such events, and routinely respond to them. Human beings, however, due to our more sophisticated brain structure, have an astounding proclivity for overriding these primitive responses. Thus, whereas animals are fairly quick to recover from potentially traumatic encounters, we are not. Whether or not a person will be traumatized depends largely on the individual's ability to respond to a threatening event in a specific way, with specific results.

When the reptilian brain perceives danger, it activates an extraordinary amount of energy—a phenomenon akin to an "adrenaline rush." This, in turn, triggers a pounding heart and other bodily changes designed to give the organism every advantage it needs to defend itself. The catch is that *to avoid being traumatized, the organism must use up all the energy that has been mobilized to deal with the threat.* Whatever energy is not discharged does not simply go away; instead, it lingers, creating the potential for a traumatic reaction to occur. The fewer resources the organism has to meet the situation, the more undischarged energy there will be, and the greater the likelihood that trauma symptoms will develop in the future.

In short, an untraumatized outcome to a threatening situation depends on one's ability to remain engaged in action, to respond effectively, and to *discharge the energy that has been mobilized,* thereby allowing the nervous system to return to its accustomed level of functioning. Even life-threatening events may not be traumatic for people who can respond and process them in a natural, effective way. And although anyone—regardless of strength, capability, or experience—can be traumatized by a threatening event, those at greatest risk are infants and children.

HOW TO TELL IF YOUR CHILD HAS BEEN TRAUMATIZED

Any unusual behavior that begins shortly after a severely frightening episode may indicate that your child is traumatized. Compulsive, repetitive mannerisms—such as repeatedly zooming a toy car into a doll —are an almost sure sign of an unresolved reaction to a traumatic event. (The activity may or may not be a literal replay of the trauma.) Other signs of traumatic stress include persistent controlling behaviors, tantrums, uncontrollable rage attacks, hyperactivity, an exaggerated startle reflex, recurring night terrors or nightmares, thrashing while asleep, bedwetting, inability to concentrate in school, forgetfulness, excessive belligerence or shyness, withdrawal or fearfulness, extreme clinginess, and stomachaches or other ailments of unknown origin.

To find out whether an uncustomary behavior is indeed a traumatic reaction, try mentioning the frightening episode and see how your child responds. A traumatized child will not want to be reminded of the predisposing event—or conversely, once reminded, will become excited or fearful and unable to stop talking about it. A traumatized child may also respond with silence.

Reminders are revealing retrospectively as well. Children who have "outgrown" unusual behavior patterns have not necessarily discharged the energy that gave rise to them. In fact, the reason traumatic reactions can hide for years is that the maturing nervous system is able to control the excess energy. By reminding your child of a frightening incident that precipitated altered behavior in years past, you may well stir up signs of traumatic residue.

Reactivating a traumatic symptom need not be cause for concern. The physiological processes involved, primitive as they are, respond well to interventions that both engage them and allow them to follow their natural course of healing. Children are wonderfully receptive to experiencing the healing side of a traumatic reaction. Your job is simply to provide an opportunity for this to occur.

RESOLVING A TRAUMATIC REACTION

Creating opportunities for healing is similar to learning the customs of a new country. It is not difficult—just different. It requires you and your child to shift from the realm of thought or emotion to the much more basic realm of *physical sensation,* where the primary task is to pay attention to how things feel and how the body is responding (*see* First Aid for Accidents and Falls on the following page). Right opportunity, in short, revolves around sensation.

A traumatized child who is in touch with internal sensations is paying attention to impulse from the reptilian core. As a result, the youngster is likely to notice subtle changes and responses, all of which are designed to help discharge excess energy and to complete feelings and responses that were previously blocked. Noticing these changes and responses enhances them.

First Aid for Accidents and Falls

Accidents and falls are a normal and often benign part of growing up. Occasionally, however, they may place a child at risk for developing a traumatic reaction. Witnessing a mishap of this sort will not necessarily clue you in to its degree of severity. For one thing, a child can be traumatized by events that seem insignificant to an adult; for another, signs of traumatic impact can be easily covered up by a child who believes that "not being hurt" will keep Mommy or Daddy happy. Your best ally in responding to your child's needs is an informed perspective.

Here are some guidelines:

- **Attend to your own responses first.** Establish a sense of calm. Being overly emotional or smothering may frighten your child at least as much as the accident itself.

- **Keep your child still and quiet.** Should injuries require that your child be moved, support or carry him, even if he appears to be able to move on his own. (A child who shows his strength may be denying the fear he feels.)

- **Encourage a sufficient interlude of safety and rest.** Help your child know what to do by being relaxed, quiet, and still yourself. If you hold him, do so in a gentle, nonrestricting way. Gently placing a hand on the center of his back, behind his heart, can communicate support and reassurance. Excessive patting or rocking is unnecessary and may interrupt the recovery process.

- **As the dazed look begins to wear off, gently guide your child's attention to his sensations**. Softly ask him how he feels "in his body." Slowly and quietly, repeat his answer as a question — "You feel OK in your body?" — and wait for a nod or other response. Be a little more specific with your next question: "How do you feel in your tummy (head, arm, leg)?" If he mentions a distinct sensation, gently ask about its location, size, shape, color, weight. In response to his answer, gently guide him to the present moment: "How does the lump (hurt, 'owie,' rock, fire) feel *now*?"

- **Allow a minute or two of silence between questions.** This will permit any cycle that may be coming through to come to completion before your child's attention is broken by another question.

- **Do not stir up discussion about the accident.** Now is the time for rest and discharge. There will be plenty of time to discuss the accident later.

- **Validate your child's physical responses.** Children often begin to cry or tremble as they come out of shock. *Resist the impulse to stop the crying or trembling.* The physical expression of distress needs to continue until it stops on its own or at least levels out, which may take only a minute. Studies have shown that children who cry after an accident have fewer problems recovering from it. As a parent, your task is to let the child know that crying and trembling are normal, healthy reactions. Place a reassuring hand on his back or shoulder, along with a statement such as, "That's OK." *The key is to avoid disrupting the responses by shifting your child's position, distracting his attention, holding him too tightly, or positioning yourself too far away to make him feel safe.*

- **Finally, attend to your child's emotional responses.** Once he appears safe and calm, encourage him to tell his experience of what happened. He may be feeling anger, fear, sadness, embarrassment, or guilt. Let your child know that whatever he is feeling is OK and worth paying attention to.

  While applying these first-aid measures, try not to be overwhelmed by worries about "doing it right." Trauma that cannot be prevented can be cured, because trauma is an *interrupted process* that is *naturally inclined to move toward completion whenever it is able to.*

The changes can be extremely subtle: something that feels internally like a rock, for example, may suddenly seem to melt into a warm liquid. *These changes have their most beneficial effect when they are simply watched, and not interpreted.* Attaching meaning to them or telling a story about them at this time may shift the child's perceptions into a more evolved portion of the brain, which can easily disrupt the direct connection established with the reptilian core.

Bodily responses that emerge along with sensations typically include involuntary trembling, shaking, and crying. If suppressed or interrupted by beliefs about being strong (grown up, courageous), acting normal, or abiding by familiar feelings, these responses will not be able to effectively discharge the accumulated energy.

Another feature of the level of experience generated by the reptilian core is the importance of rhythm and timing. Think about it . . . everything in the wild is dictated by cycles. The seasons turn, the moon waxes and wanes, tides come in and go out, the sun rises and sets. Animals follow the rhythms of nature—mating, birthing, feeding, hunting, sleeping, and hibernating in direct response to nature's pendulum. So too, do the responses that bring natural traumatic reactions to their natural resolution.

For human beings, these rhythms pose a two-fold challenge. First, they move at a much slower pace than we are accustomed to. And second, they are entirely beyond our control. *Healing cycles can only be opened up to, watched, and validated; they cannot be evaluated, manipulated, hurried, or changed.* When they do not get the time and attention they need, they are rarely able to complete their healing mission.

Immersed in the realm of instinctual responses, your child will undergo at least one such cycle. How can you tell when it is complete? Tune in to your child. Traumatized children who remain in the sensing mode without engaging their thought processes, *feel a release and an opening;* their attention then focuses back on the external world. You will be able to sense this shift in your child, and know that a healing has occurred.

Resolving a traumatic reaction does much more than eliminate the likelihood of reactions emerging later in life. It fosters, in essence, a *natural resilience to stress.* Certainly, a nervous system accustomed to moving into stress and then out of it is far healthier than a nervous system burdened with an ongoing, if not accumulating, level of stress. And just as certainly, children who are encouraged to attend to their instinctual responses are rewarded with a lifelong legacy of health and vigor.

The information in this section has been reprinted from "Understanding Childhood Trauma" and "First Aid for Accidents and Falls" by Peter Levine, Ph.D. It has been reprinted with permission. Dr. Levine, who holds doctorates in medical biophysics and psychology, has been working in the area of stress and trauma for over twenty-five years. Dr. Levine is also the author of *Waking the Tiger—Healing Trauma Through the Body.*

For information regarding the social and global impacts of trauma, write: The Foundation for Human Enrichment, PO Box 1872, Lyons, CO 80540. For further information about books, articles, public lectures, or professional training programs in the field of trauma, contact: Ergos Institute for Somatic Education, PO Box 110, Lyons, CO 80540; (303) 823–9524.

Part Two

Life-Saving Techniques and Procedures

Introduction

Being prepared in a time of crisis is the best way to maintain a much-needed calm, clear head. An emergency situation is likely to elicit panic from both the parent and child. As a responsible caregiver, you would be wise to familiarize yourself with the following life-saving techniques and procedures. Knowing what to do when an emergency arises can help to possibly save a life.

Steps for initiating cardiopulmonary resuscitation (CPR), should your child stop breathing, are presented in this section, as well as guidelines for performing first aid for choking in the event your child has a piece of food or another object lodged in his throat and is unable to breathe. The Heimlich maneuver, named for its developer Dr. H. J. Heimlich, for both infants under one year old and children over one year are outlined.

In the event your child sustains a broken bone or a serious injury to his neck, head, or back, emergency procedures for immobilizing these areas are offered in this section, as well as the proper way to apply a pressure bandage to stop severe bleeding. And in a further effort to keep you—a responsible caregiver—informed and prepared, important conventional diagnostic techniques are also provided. These include entries that outline the correct procedures for taking your child's temperature and pulse.

The techniques and procedures presented in Part Two are not meant to teach you everything in a time of crisis, but are to be used as refreshers for a course on emergency first aid that includes CPR for infants and children, and instruction in the Heimlich maneuver. We strongly recommend that anyone who cares for a child on a regular basis obtains such hands-on training. Courses are available through the Red Cross and many local hospitals.

First Aid for Choking

If a child with something stuck in her throat is talking or coughing forcefully, it means that air is getting through the windpipe and you don't need to interfere. As long as she can breathe, she may be able to expel the material without help. But if your child is unable to speak, making high-pitched sounds or gasping for air, turning blue, or clutching at her throat, have someone call for emergency help, while you go to your child's aid quickly.

Follow the directions below in the manner appropriate for your child's age. Please note that the information in this entry is not meant to serve as a substitute for a hands-on course in first aid, but as a review should you ever be called upon to use your first aid training. Emergency first aid courses are offered through the Red Cross and many local hospitals.

For a Choking Infant Under One Year Old

The Heimlich maneuver should be performed on an infant under one year old as follows:

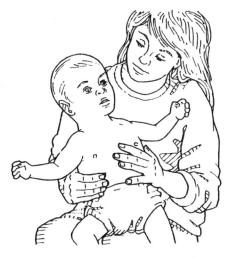

1. Sit on a chair and place your baby on your lap facing away from you.

For a Choking Child Over One Year Old

The Heimlich maneuver should be performed on a child over one year old as follows:

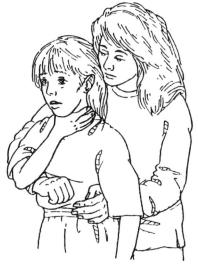

1. Stand or kneel behind your child, wrapping your arms around her waist.

29

For a Choking Infant Under One Year Old

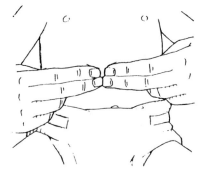

2. Put the tips of both of your index and middle fingers together to form one compression pad. Position this "pad" against your baby's abdomen, above the navel and just below the rib cage.

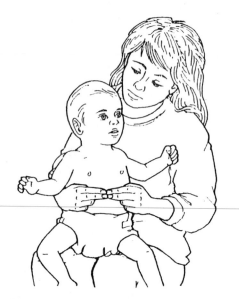

3. Use a gentle, quick, *upward* push into your baby's abdomen to force air up through the windpipe.

4. Continue doing these thrusts until your baby expels the foreign material.

For a Choking Child Over One Year Old

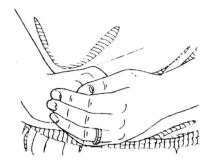

2. Make a fist with one hand and clasp your other hand over your fist. Position the thumb side of your fist against your child's abdomen, above the navel and just below the rib cage.

3. Use a quick, forceful, *upward* push of your fist into your child's abdomen to force air up through the windpipe.

4. Continue doing these thrusts until your child expels the foreign material.

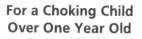

For a Choking Infant
Under One Year Old

If your baby loses consciousness at any time, discontinue the thrusts and open her airway as follows:

5. Look for foreign material in your baby's mouth. If you see anything, remove it, but **do not** blindly sweep your finger through the infant's mouth.

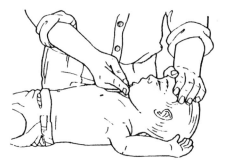

6. Tip your baby's head back by pushing on her forehead. With your other hand, gently lift the bony part of the jaw. This positioning opens the airway.

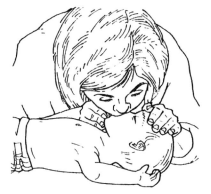

7. Cover your baby's nose and mouth with your mouth and give 2 gentle puffs of air, just enough to make her chest rise and fall as in normal breathing.

For a Choking Child
Over One Year Old

If your child loses consciousness at any time, discontinue the thrusts and open her airway as follows:

5. Place your child on her back. Look for foreign material in her mouth. If you see anything, remove it, but **do not** blindly sweep your finger through her mouth.

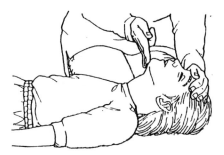

6. Tip your child's head back by pushing on her forehead. With your other hand, gently lift the bony part of the jaw. This positioning opens the airway.

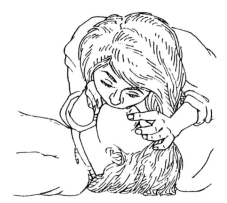

7. Pinch your child's nostrils closed. Cover her mouth with yours and give 2 slow breaths of air, enough to make her chest rise and fall as in normal breathing.

For a Choking Infant Under One Year Old

If your baby's chest is not rising and falling when you give the breaths, her airway is still blocked. You will have to try again to dislodge the foreign material.

8. Repeat steps 1 through 4 until the material is expelled, *or* your baby begins coughing, breathing, and making normal sounds on her own, *or* another person can take over for you, *or* emergency help arrives.

For a Choking Child Over One Year Old

If your child's chest is not rising and falling when you give the breaths, her airway is still blocked. You will have to try again to dislodge the foreign material.

8. Repeat steps 1 through 4 until the material is expelled, *or* your child begins coughing, breathing, and making normal sounds on her own, *or* another person can take over for you, *or* emergency help arrives.

Even if your child seems to be fine once the material has been expelled, she should be seen by a doctor to be checked for possible damage to her windpipe or abdomen. For additional information on emergency treatment for choking, *see* CHOKING in Part Three.

Cardiopulmonary Resuscitation (CPR)

The following emergency procedures can sustain life if a child's breathing and/or heart have stopped. When respiration stops, the body begins to be deprived of oxygen, which can cause serious damage. Brain cells begin to die within four to six minutes if they are deprived of oxygen. Cardiopulmonary resuscitation (CPR) keeps blood and oxygen circulating in the body. By breathing into your child's lungs and pressing on his heart, you can maintain blood flow and oxygen/carbon dioxide exchange to the brain and other organs until he recovers or until emergency medical personnel arrive to take over.

Although the following information on administering CPR is valuable, it is best to obtain training under the guidance of a qualified instructor. Emergency first-aid courses are offered through the Red Cross and many local hospitals. Reading about the procedures cannot substitute for taking a course and practicing on a mannequin under the guidance of a qualified instructor. Further, these practices are constantly being researched and revised. Stay informed.

In addition to the usual mouth-to-mouth breathing, CPR can involve other procedures in special circumstances, such as giving CPR to a child with a potential spinal-cord injury, mouth-to-nose breathing, mouth-to-nose-and-mouth breathing (as with an infant), and mouth-to-stoma breathing (a stoma is a surgically created opening in the body, such as a tracheostomy). Only instruction and practice with a qualified instructor in attendance will adequately prepare you to give CPR.

If your child loses consciousness, is not breathing, and/or loses his pulse, assess the situation quickly, call for emergency help, and initiate CPR in the following manner that is appropriate to the child's age.

CPR for an Infant Under One Year Old

OPEN THE AIRWAY

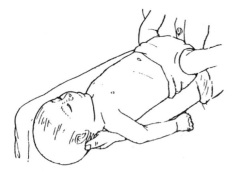

1. Hold your baby securely in the crook of your arm, face up.

2. Look for any foreign material in your baby's mouth. If you see anything, remove it with your finger. **Do not** blindly sweep your finger through your child's mouth.

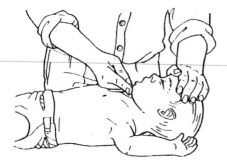

3. Tip your baby's head back by pushing on her forehead. With your other hand, gently lift the bony part of the jaw. This positioning opens the airway.

CPR for a Child Over One Year Old

OPEN THE AIRWAY

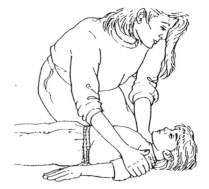

1. Place your child on her back on the floor.

2. Look for any foreign material in your child's mouth. If you see anything, remove it with your finger. **Do not** blindly sweep your finger through your child's mouth.

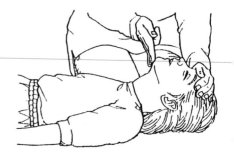

3. Tip your child's head back by pushing on her forehead. With your other hand, gently lift the bony part of the jaw. This positioning opens the airway.

CPR for an Infant Under One Year Old

CPR for a Child Over One Year Old

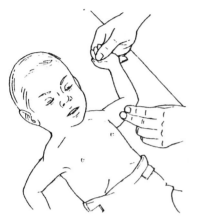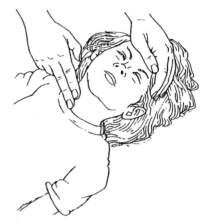

4. Check for a pulse on the brachial artery by placing the tips of your first two fingers on your child's inner arm above the elbow (see above).

5. Check for breathing by putting your cheek close to the baby's mouth to feel for a breath, and watch her chest to see if it is rising and falling as in normal breathing.

If the baby is not breathing on her own, take steps to restore breathing (see step 6). If there is no pulse, initiate full CPR (go to step 9).

4. Check for a pulse on the carotid artery, located at the side of the neck. Touch your first two fingers to the Adam's apple. Run your fingers across the neck to the depression between the Adam's apple and the large neck muscle (see above). Press gently.

5. Check for breathing by putting your cheek close to your child's mouth to feel for a breath, and watch her chest to see if it is rising and falling as in normal breathing.

If your child is not breathing on her own, take steps to restore breathing (see step 6). If there is no pulse, initiate full CPR (go to step 9).

CPR for an Infant Under One Year Old	CPR for a Child Over One Year Old

RESTORE BREATHING	**RESTORE BREATHING**

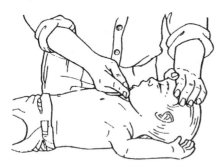 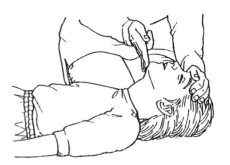

6. Again, tip your baby's head back by pushing on her forehead. With your other hand, gently lift the bony part of the jaw. This positioning opens the airway.

6. Again, tip your child's head back by pushing on her forehead. With your other hand, gently lift the bony part of the jaw. This positioning opens the airway.

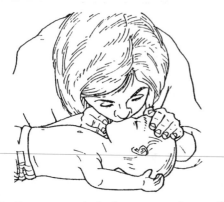 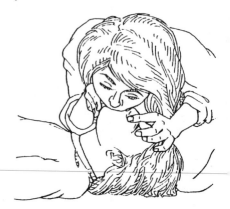

7. Cover your baby's nose and mouth with your mouth and give 2 gentle puffs of air, just enough to make your baby's chest rise and fall as in normal breathing. Watch to see if your child's chest is rising and falling when you give breaths. If it isn't, repeat steps 1 through 3 and give 2 more puffs of air.

7. Pinch your child's nostrils closed Cover her mouth with yours and give 2 slow breaths of air. Watch to see if your child's chest is rising and falling as in normal breathing. If it isn't, repeat steps 1 through 3 and give 2 more puffs of air.

CPR for an Infant
Under One Year Old

CPR for a Child
Over One Year Old

8. If your baby is still not breathing, the airway may be blocked. If you suspect choking, immediately turn to page 29 and perform steps 1 through 4 to expel the foreign material.

If your baby loses her pulse during this procedure, immediately initiate full CPR (see step 9)

8. If your child is still not breathing, the airway may be blocked. If you suspect choking, immediately turn to page 29 and perform steps 1 through 4 to expel the foreign material.

If your child loses her pulse during this procedure, immediately initiate full CPR (see step 9).

FULL CPR

FULL CPR

9. Place your baby flat on the floor on her back. Check for a pulse on her brachial artery again (step 4). Only if your child's heart has stopped beating and you cannot feel a pulse can you safely begin CPR.

Never do chest compressions on a child with a heartbeat.

9. Place your child flat on the floor on her back. Check for a pulse on her carotid artery again (step 4). Only if your child's heart has stopped beating and you cannot feel a pulse can you safely begin CPR.

Never do chest compressions on a child with a heartbeat.

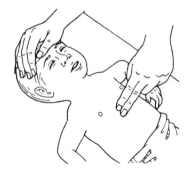

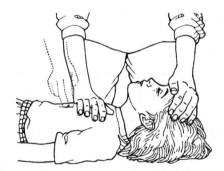

10. If your baby *is not* breathing and *does not* have a pulse, give compressions. Locate the spot to give compressions by placing two or three fingers on her chest just below the nipple line (*see* above).

10. If your child *is not* breathing and *does not* have a pulse, give compressions. Place your middle finger on the notch where the ribs and sternum meet. Put your index finger next to your middle finger (*see* above). Place the heel of your hand right next to the index finger (*see* above). Straddle your child.

CPR for an Infant Under One Year Old

CPR for a Child Over One Year Old

11. Keep your elbows straight and your shoulders aligned over your baby's body. Maintain this position so that the compressions are done straight up and down on your baby's chest.

12. For each compression, push your baby's breastbone down with your fingers the equivalent of a third to half of her total chest height (approximately $\frac{1}{2}$ to 1 inch) straight down. **Do not** rock your body. **Do not** move into your child's chest diagonally. Release the pressure between compressions without taking your fingers off her chest.

13. Perform cycles of chest compressions and respirations. A complete cycle consists of at least 5 chest compressions followed by 1 breath. Give at least 20 breaths per minute (1 breath every 3 seconds) and 100 compressions per minute.

Count aloud to help maintain a steady rhythm: One one-thousand, two one-thousand, three one-thousand, four one-thousand, five one-thousand, and BREATH, and so on.

14. After giving CPR for one minute, check your baby's brachial pulse again (step 4). If you feel a pulse, stop doing chest compressions and check for breathing.

15. If there is still no pulse, continue performing chest compressions, while checking for a pulse and breathing every few minutes. **Do not** stop CPR until your baby starts breathing on her own, *or* another person can take over for you, *or* emergency help arrives.

11. Keep your elbows straight and your shoulders aligned over your child's body. Maintain this position so that the compressions are done straight up and down on your child's chest.

12. For each compression, push your child's breastbone down with the heel of your hand the equivalent of a third to half of her total chest height (approximately 1 to $1\frac{1}{2}$ inches) straight down. **Do not** rock your body. **Do not** move into your child's chest diagonally. Release the pressure between compressions without taking the heel of your hand off her chest.

13. Perform cycles of chest compressions and respirations. A complete cycle consists of 5 chest compressions followed by 1 breath. Give 20 breaths per minute (1 breath every 3 seconds) and 100 compressions per minute.

Count aloud to help maintain a steady rhythm: One one-thousand, two one-thousand, three one-thousand, four one-thousand, five one-thousand, and BREATH, and so on.

14. After giving CPR for one minute, check your child's carotid pulse again (step 4). If you feel a pulse, stop doing chest compressions and check for breathing.

15. If there is still no pulse, continue performing chest compressions while checking for a pulse and breathing every few minutes. **Do not** stop CPR until your child starts breathing on her own, *or* another person can take over for you, *or* emergency help arrives.

CPR for an Infant Under One Year Old	CPR for a Child Over One Year Old
16. If your baby begins breathing on her own, discontinue CPR. Once her pulse and breathing have been restored, and the immediate crisis is over, check and treat your baby for bleeding, broken bones, or any other injury or problem she might have.	**16.** If your child begins breathing on her own, discontinue CPR. Once her pulse and breathing have been restored, and the immediate crisis is over, check and treat your baby for bleeding, broken bones, or any other injury or problem she might have.

Immobilizing a Broken Bone

If your child has suffered an accident, a bad fall, or a hard blow, he may have broken a bone. A broken bone is painful at the site of the break and may appear swollen, red, and bruised. The affected limb may look crooked or bent, or there may be an open wound at the fracture site. Depending on which bone is broken, there is a possibility of further damage, including internal bleeding. A broken rib may puncture a lung; a broken vertebra can damage the spinal cord; a skull fracture can cause bleeding into the skull. Broken bones must be taken seriously and treated immediately.

If you think your child may have suffered a bone fracture of any kind, *do not attempt to straighten the bone.* Further movement can cause additional injury to the nerves, tissues, and arteries. As a child's bones are still growing, it is critical that any fracture be treated appropriately by a qualified professional. *If you suspect your child has a broken or injured neck, back, or skull, turn immediately to page 44.*

Although the following information provided on immobilizing broken bones is valuable and helpful during emergency situations, it is best to learn and practice these guidelines under the expertise of a qualified instructor. Taking an emergency first aid course through the Red Cross or a local hospital is the best preparation. (For more information, *see* BONES, BROKEN in Part Three)

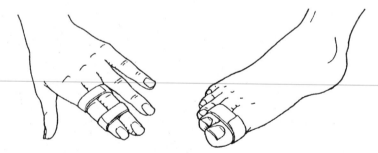

✚ Immobilizing a Finger or Toe:

1. Place a cotton ball or a small piece of cloth between the injured finger or toe and an uninjured one. Tape them together. (Do this only if it does not cause further pain.)
2. Apply cold compresses.

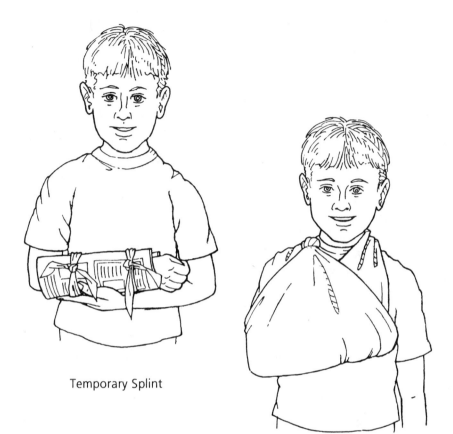

Temporary Splint

A Sling

✚ Immobilizing a Broken Forearm, Wrist, or Hand:

1. While carefully supporting the injured area, place the child's forearm at a right angle over his stomach. Using a magazine or section of newspaper as a temporary splint, wrap up the entire forearm. Tie up the "splint" on either side of the injury, making sure it fits snugly, but not so tight that it cuts off circulation. (Use this same splint technique to immobilize an injured upper arm.)

2. To make a sling, fold a large piece of cloth to form a triangle—you can use a towel, shirt, sweater, etc. Place the wide part of the triangle under the injured forearm. Bring the two ends of the cloth around the child's neck and tie them together.

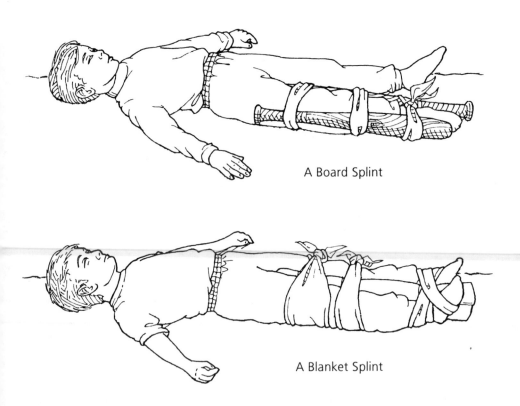

A Board Splint

A Blanket Splint

✚ Immobilizing a Broken Lower Leg:

You can make a temporary splint for a broken lower leg out of either two boards or a blanket.

1. For a board splint, you'll need two boards or poles (mop or broomstick handles or even baseball bats will do). One board should be the length of your child's leg from his hip to his foot. The other board should extend from your child's groin area to his foot. Pad the boards with towels or other soft cloths and place them snugly on both sides of the broken leg. Tie the boards in place at the waist, thigh, knee, and ankle.

2. For a blanket splint, place a rolled-up blanket between your child's legs, then tie his legs together at the thighs, knees, and ankles.

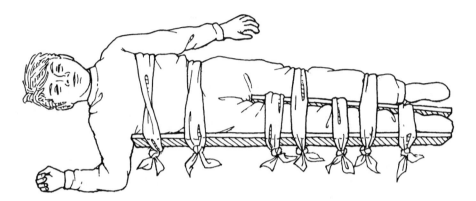

✚ Immobilizing a Broken Upper Leg or Hip:

Do not attempt to splint a broken upper leg or hip unless the child has to be moved. During such emergency situations, however, when it is necessary to make a splint, do the following:

1. First, you will need two boards or poles (mop or broomstick handles or even baseball bats will do). One board should be the length of your child's armpit to his foot. The other should extend from his groin to his foot.

2. Pad the boards with towels or other soft cloths and place them snugly on both sides of the leg.

3. Tie the boards in place at the chest, waist, groin, thigh, knee, and ankle.

Immobilizing an Injured Head, Neck, and Back

Any additional movement to an injured head, neck, or back can cause further damage. If your child has sustained such an injury, *do not move him unless it is absolutely necessary* (such as when facing a life-or-death situation—an impending explosion, fire, or other peril). While waiting for help to arrive, it is important to immobilize the child's head and neck, and possibly his entire body, to prevent further movement.

Although the following immobilization techniques are valuable and helpful during emergency situations, it is best to learn and practice these guidelines under the expertise of a qualified instructor. Taking an emergency first aid course through the Red Cross or a local hospital is the best preparation. (For more information, *see* BONES, BROKEN in Part Three.)

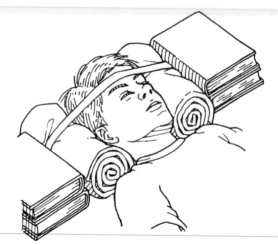

✚ Immobilizing an Injured Head and/or Neck:

1. Without moving or elevating the child, place two rolled-up towels or blankets an either side of his head. If possible, tape his head to the floor.

2. Firmly secure the towels with heavy objects such as books, bricks, or heavy boxes.

3. If transferring the child is absolutely necessary, be sure to move his entire body in one motion as a unit (without twisting the torso).

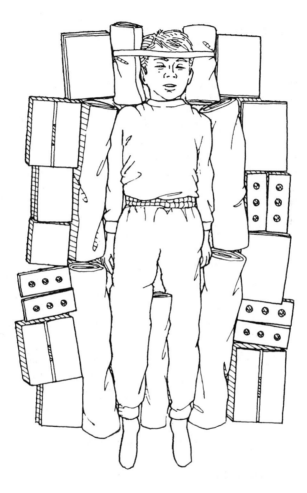

✚ Immobilizing the Entire Body:

1. After immobilizing the child's head and neck (as on page 44), place more rolled-up towels or blankets along the sides of his body.

2. Firmly secure the towels with heavy objects such as books, bricks, or heavy boxes.

3. If transferring the child is absolutely necessary, be sure to move his entire body in one motion as a unit (without twisting the torso).

Applying a Pressure Bandage

If your child is bleeding severely from an external wound, do the following:

1. Cover the bleeding wound with a clean cloth or gauze and quickly apply very firm, steady pressure. If there is no clean cloth or gauze immediately available, use your bare hand to apply pressure. Even if your child complains that it hurts, continue applying firm, steady pressure. It is necessary to stop the bleeding. If the wound has a foreign object, such as a piece of glass or wood, be careful not to push it further into the wound with your pressure.

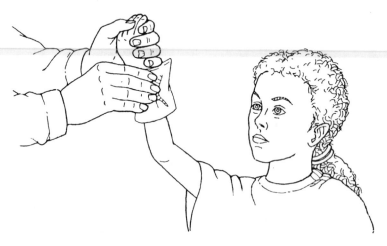

Raising the Wound Above Heart Level

2. If there is no suspicion of a spinal injury, raise the wound above the level of the heart to help minimize the amount of blood that spurts from the wound with every heartbeat. Signs of a spinal injury include pain at the site of the injury, weakness or numbness in an extremity, inability to move an extremity, or lack of feeling in an extremity. If any of these signs are present, **do not** move your child. If you do, you may worsen the injury.

3. If blood soaks through the cloth pad or gauze, put more cloth or gauze over the old pad and continue applying pressure. Do not remove the original blood-soaked pad. Early clotting may become dislodged.

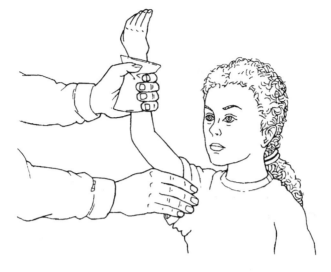

Applying Additional Pressure to Pressure Points

4. If steady pressure and elevation cannot control the bleeding, place additional pressure with your fingers and thumb on the pressure point that is closest to the injury and between the injury and the heart (*see* above). If the femoral artery, located in the groin area, is to be compressed, use the heel of your hand. (*See* figure on page 48 for location of pressure points.)

5. If emergency medical personnel are not on their way to you, take your child to the nearest emergency room. If you have another adult with you, have that person see to the transportation while you hold your child and continue applying pressure. If you are alone and must drive, tie the cloth or gauze firmly in place to maintain pressure on the wound. Check for a pulse beat below the cloth to make sure the tissues are receiving adequate blood.

6. A tourniquet is a bandage that is tied so tightly that it cuts off the flow of blood to an area of the body, usually a portion of an arm or a leg. It is a drastic measure that is appropriate only if blood loss is so severe and rapid as to be immediately life threatening. ***Do not apply a tourniquet unless it is absolutely necessary, and then only as a last resort.*** Because a tourniquet cuts off blood, it deprives the tissues below the wound of oxygen, creating the risk of your child losing a limb. If your child is losing so much blood so rapidly that you must put on a tourniquet, be sure to mark it with the time the tourniquet was applied. Never cover a tourniquet. It is vital that medical personnel can see immediately that a tourniquet is in place.

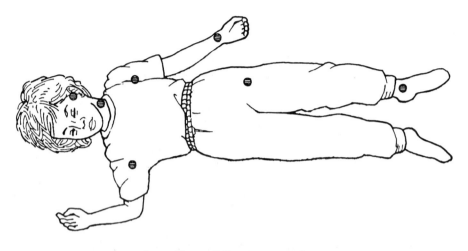

Location of Pressure Points

A severe loss of blood will cause shock, which can be life threatening. Try to remain calm and reassuring. Any panic you display will be transmitted to your child and make the situation worse. Your immediate task is to stem the flow of blood and secure emergency medical care for your child.

Do not give your child any medicine, food, or liquid of any kind before a doctor has assessed the situation. It is important that your child's stomach be empty, as surgery may be needed to repair the wound.

For additional information on treatment for severe external bleeding, *see* BLEEDING, SEVERE in Part Three.

Taking Your Child's Temperature

Normal body temperature probably has a much wider range than previously thought. No longer is 98.6°F considered standard. Temperature also varies throughout the day. In general, any oral temperature above 101°F is considered elevated. However, except for infants less than two months old, it is not usually necessary to treat a temperature under 102°F unless it is making your child uncomfortable.

There are a number of different ways to take a child's temperature: orally, rectally, and under the arm. The way you choose will be determined by your child's age and by her ability to keep still for three minutes or so. In addition to standard mercury thermometers, there are now digital thermometers available that can take a child's temperature in much less time. These are convenient if you have a child who is squirmy and uncomfortable. Another option that is more expensive but not as reliable is a device that measures temperature in the ear. If the ear is clogged with wax or the device is not properly positioned in the ear, this type of thermometer will register an inaccurate reading. Another device that measures temperature is the forehead strip. It is the opinion of the authors that these strips are simply not reliable in determining a child's temperature. Ask your nurse or doctor which type or types he or she considers the most reliable.

Regardless of which method you choose, *never* leave any child alone with a thermometer. Also, if you notice a crack in the thermometer, throw it out. The mercury it contains is poisonous.

If your child has just eaten or drunk something warm or cold, is dressed very warmly, or has just been exercising, wait thirty minutes before taking her temperature to be sure you get an accurate reading.

ORAL METHOD

If your child is older than five years, you can take her temperature orally.

1. Wash the thermometer with cool water, then shake it down so that it registers less than 96°F.

2. Place the silver or red end of the thermometer under your child's tongue or along the inside of her cheek. Either you or your child can hold it in place. Don't let your child use her teeth to hold it there.

DEGREES FAHRENHEIT TO CENTIGRADE

98.6°F = 37°C	103°F = 39.5°C
99.5°F = 37.5°C	104°F = 40°C
100°F = 37.8°C	105°F = 40.6°C
100.4°F = 38°C	106°F = 41.1°C
101°F = 38.4°C	107°F = 41.7°C
102°F = 38.9°C	

3. Leave the thermometer in place for at least three minutes before removing it.

4. After reading your child's temperature, wash the thermometer with cool water, then clean it with isopropyl rubbing alcohol.

RECTAL METHOD

Because young children are so active, and because babies and younger children cannot hold a thermometer in their mouths, a rectal temperature may be your best (and only) option. To take your child's temperature rectally, you will need a rectal thermometer, which has a round bulb at the end. Be aware that a rectal temperature is usually about 0.8°F higher than an oral temperature.

1. Wash the thermometer with cool water, then shake it down so that it registers less than 96°F.

2. Dip the bulb end of the thermometer in petroleum jelly, and gently insert it about one inch into your baby's rectum.

3. Hold the thermometer in place for three minutes before removing it. It is a good idea to have a towel or washcloth on hand in case of an "accident" when removing the thermometer.

4. After reading your child's temperature, wash the thermometer with cool water, then clean it with isopropyl rubbing alcohol.

UNDERARM METHOD

If your child is under five years old or unable to hold a thermometer in her mouth, you can try to take her temperature under the arm. This method usually yields a temperature reading that is approximately 1°F lower than an oral temperature. Because it does not always give as reliable a reading as the other methods do, it is best used only as a general indicator.

1. Wash the thermometer with cool water, then shake it down so that it registers less than 96°F.

2. Place the silver or red end of the thermometer under your child's armpit. Make sure the armpit is dry before placing the thermometer.

3. Leave the thermometer in place for three minutes before removing it.

4. After reading your child's temperature, wash the thermometer with cool water, then clean it with isopropyl rubbing alcohol.

Taking Your Child's Pulse

Taking your child's pulse is a diagnostic procedure that is easily performed. Different techniques are recommended for children under and over one year of age, as outlined below.

For an Infant Under One Year Old

To take the pulse of an infant less than one year old, feel for a pulse at the brachial artery, the artery that carries blood to the arm.

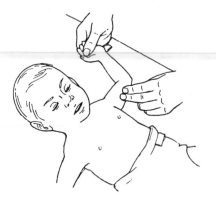

1. Place the tips of your first two fingers on your infant's inner arm above the elbow. Feel the pulse at the brachial artery.

2. Using a precise timer, such as the second hand of your watch, count the number of pulses you feel for one minute, or count the pulses for ten seconds and multiply by six.

3. Another place you can feel for a pulse is at the femoral artery, which is located at the groin.

For a Child Over One Year Old

To take the pulse of a child over one year old, feel for a pulse at the carotid artery, located on the side of the neck.

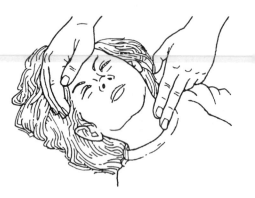

1. Touch your first two fingers to your child's Adam's apple, then run your fingers across her neck to the depression between the Adam's apple and the large neck muscle. Feel the pulse at the carotid artery.

2. Using a precise timer, such as the second hand of your watch, count the number of pulses you feel for one minute, or count the pulses for ten seconds and multiply by six.

3. Another place you can feel for a pulse is at the radial artery, which is located on the thumb side of the wrist.

Part Three
The Emergencies

Introduction

Accidents and emergency situations can—and do—happen, even in the most careful and well-prepared households. Knowing what to do when the unthinkable occurs can literally mean the difference between life and death for your child.

Part Three begins with a small section that includes basic guidelines to follow when faced with an emergency, as well as some general information about the emergency entries themselves. What follows is an A-to-Z listing of common medical emergency situations you may encounter with your child. Each entry contains an explanation of the problem, followed by an emergency treatment procedure. Depending on the nature of the emergency, some entries include preventive measures and other general recommendations.

Emergency Situations

We strongly recommend that the primary child-care provider in the family (as well as anyone else who cares for children on a regular basis) complete a good hands-on course in emergency first aid that includes CPR for infants and children, and instructions for other emergency procedures. There is simply no substitute for the instruction and practice you will get in a good first aid course.

The following are general guidelines to follow in responding to any emergency, no matter what its nature.

☐ *Stay calm. Take a moment to assess what has happened.* It won't help your child if you scream or panic. Your child needs you to be a calm and reassuring presence.

☐ *Make sure your child is breathing and check for a pulse.* Check for breathing by putting your cheek close to your child's mouth to feel for a breath, and watch his chest to see if it is rising and falling as in normal breathing. For an infant under one year, check for a pulse on the brachial artery by placing the tips of your first two fingers on the infant's inner arm above the elbow. For a child older than one year, check for a pulse on the carotid artery, located at the side of the neck. Touch your first two fingers to the Adam's apple, and run your fingers across the neck to the depression between the Adam's apple and the large neck muscle. Allow five to ten seconds to feel for a pulse. If your child is not breathing or does not have a pulse, turn to CARDIOPULMONARY RESUSCITATION (CPR) on page 33. Begin performing CPR at once.

☐ *Check for bleeding and for obviously broken bones.*

☐ *Try to determine what has happened.* If your child can respond, ask. If not, observe the surroundings. For example, is there a bottle of pills or cleaning compounds nearby? Is the child lying on her back under a tree? If the person is unknown to you, is she wearing a Medic Alert bracelet that identifies a specific medical condition? The few moments you take to assess the situation are vitally important. After close observation, you'll have a better sense of whom to call and what to do. Without careful assessment, you are more likely to panic and do the wrong thing.

☐ *If you suspect a head, neck, or spinal injury, do not pick up or move the child, even to offer comfort.* Moving someone with a possible head, neck, or back injury can worsen the damage. Unless there is a threat that the child will vomit and choke, it is best to leave her in the same position in which you found her. Rely on medical personnel to know how to stabilize the child so that transport to the hospital will be safe.

☐ *Call for emergency help.* When calling for emergency help, speak distinctly. Give your name, the address you're calling from, your phone number, and your assessment of the situation. *Don't rush.* If you remain calm, you will save time in the long run. If you give clear, distinct, precise information so that the operator can route emergency help to your location quickly, you won't have to repeat your message. Try to relate enough of the problem so that the people who respond to your call will be prepared to deal with it when they arrive. You don't have to know exactly what's wrong; just convey as clearly and completely as you can what you have observed and what your assessment of the situation is.

☐ *Stay with your child.* Try to stay with your child until emergency personnel arrive, or until the situation is resolved. If possible, have someone else place the call for emergency services. Your child needs to feel the reassurance of your presence. Talk to her, using simple explanations to describe what's happening. Fear of the unknown makes matters worse. If you are sure that she has not suffered an injury to her head, neck, or back, hold your child close. Otherwise, just gently touch and soothe. As you do so, carefully observe any changes in your child's condition, such as shifts in breathing or heart rate, or changes in her level of pain or consciousness. Certain emergencies will require your immediate intervention.

☐ *Be alert for signs of shock.* Shock is a serious condition that results from a sudden and life-threatening drop in blood pressure, which in turn impairs circulation and threatens the brain's oxygen supply. Shock can occur after any trauma to the body, whether from near-drowning, severe injury, major blood loss, or overwhelming infection.

A child suffering from shock may become pale and sweaty, possibly drowsy, confused, and/or disoriented. Shock is usually accompanied by profound weakness, dizziness, faintness, and a cold sweat. The pulse may be weak and feeble.

If you suspect shock, lay your child down on her back and put pillows under her feet to raise her feet higher than her head. Loosen tight or constricting clothing, and cover your child with a blanket. The goal is to insure normal breathing while maintaining normal body temperature and adequate blood circulation to the brain.

If emergency personnel are not already on their way to you, seek emergency medical attention for your child immediately.

☐ Depending on the nature of the emergency, refer to the appropriate emergency listed in this section.

ABOUT THE EMERGENCY ENTRIES

What follows is an alphabetical listing of common medical emergencies. Each individual entry contains an explanation of the problem followed by an emergency treatment procedure. For some cases, in which an emergency situation may not be obvious (for example, during bouts of excessive nausea or diarrhea), information on "when to call the doctor" is provided. Also, depending on the nature of the emergency, a number of entries include preventive measures and other general recommendations.

Certainly, modern medicine is invaluable to a child and his family in an emergency situation. Once the emergency treatment has been properly administered, however, and the child is considered stable, certain natural therapeutics—herbals and homeopathic remedies—are important in helping to further stabilize, nourish, and heal the body. Wherever appropriate, we have suggested their use under the General Recommendation section of each emergency entry. Consumers can find a wide variety of such natural products in both drugstores and health food shops. Remember, the suggested use of these remedies is to be considered only after the emergency treatment has been given. Should you have any questions concerning the appropriate use of any preparation mentioned in this book, always consult your professional health care provider before using.

A Guide to Common Symptoms

The guide below lists some of the more common symptoms children experience during emergency medical situations. It is not a comprehensive list but rather a guide that can help you when your child is not feeling well. Although your child may be experiencing one or some of the symptoms listed here, she may or may not have any of the illnesses mentioned. Diseases are listed because they can cause the particular symptoms, and they are listed in alphabetical order, not in order of the likelihood of occurrence

Among the possible causes that have been listed for each symptom, those that are **bold-faced** are emergency in nature. Listings for these emergency causes are presented in this section.

This chart is not meant to substitute for the advice of a qualified health care provider; always consult with your doctor or other practitioner for a professional diagnosis.

Symptom	Possible Causes
Abdominal pain	**Appendicitis,** bowel obstruction, colic, constipation, emotional upset, **food allergies, food poisoning, gas, internal bleeding, nausea.**
Loss of appetite	**Appendicitis,** emotional upset, infection.
Difficulty breathing	**Allergies, anaphylactic reaction, asthma, choking,** croup, **fever,** infection, **seizure, shock.**
Rapid breathing	**Allergies, asthma,** infection, **shock.**
Cold sweat	Anxiety, heart problems, infection, **internal bleeding,** intestinal disorders, **shock.**
Cough	**Allergies, asthma, choking,** infection.
Diarrhea	**Appendicitis, food poisoning,** infection.
Drowsiness	**Concussion,** dehydration, **hypothermia,** infection.
Earache	**Allergies,** fluid in ear, foreign body in ear, **head injury,** infection.
Eye inflammation	**Allergies, chemical burn, eye injury,** infection, **sunburn.**
Fever	**Appendicitis,** certain cancers, dehydration, **heat illness,** infection.
Headache	**Allergies,** altitude sickness, **concussion,** emotional upset, **meningitis,** sinus infection.

Symptom	Possible Causes
Irritability, restlessness	**Allergies, asthma,** colic, emotional upset, infection.
Aching joints	Infection (**Lyme disease,** influenza), rheumatoid arthritis, trauma.
Mouth sores	Cold sores (herpes and other viruses), **food allergies,** trauma.
Runny or stuffy nose	**Allergies** (airborne or food), common cold, sinus infection.
Seizure	Epilepsy, **fever, head injury, meningitis.**
Skin rash, lesions, or bumps	**Allergies** (food or contact), **insect bites, poison ivy, poison oak, poison sumac, sunburn,** viral illnesses (eg. chickenpox, measles)
Unconsciousness	**Concussion, fainting, severe bleeding, shock.**
Unusually widened pupils	Bleeding into the brain from trauma, **concussion,** neurological disorders, **overdose of certain drugs.**
Vomiting	Altitude sickness, **appendicitis, concussion,** emotional upset, **food allergies, food poisoning,** infection, **internal bleeding,** intestinal obstruction, motion sickness, **shock.**

As a responsible parent or caregiver, you may want to page through this section to familiarize yourself with some of the emergency situations and their treatments. In some cases, certain emergencies may be more likely to occur and, therefore, preparing yourself to deal with them beforehand is wise. For instance, if you live in an area where snakes and poisonous insects are prevalent, it would make sense for you to turn to the sections on snakebites and insect bites and stings. Acquaint yourself with how to prepare for and deal with such emergencies. Maybe you live near a body of water or have a swimming pool in your yard. For you, it would be particularly helpful to read the entry on near-drowning and learn exactly what to do in such a situation. If you live in an area that experiences unusually hot weather, the entry on heat illness may be especially useful.

Whatever your situation, it is always best to be prepared. Emergency circumstances are usually charged with emotion, often bordering on panic. Being prepared is the best way to maintain a much-needed calm, clear head. (To further prepare yourself through preventive measures, be sure to familiarize yourself with the guidelines presented in Part One, "Safety Measures."

AFTER THE EMERGENCY HAS PASSED

After emergency medical treatment or procedures have been administered, often the body is left physically weak and exhausted. Standard medicines and methods may also leave emotional scars that need to be addressed. Once the crisis is over, administering natural treatments and therapies can be significant in helping the body heal and further stabilize.

Natural Remedies Following Physical Trauma

Consider the following natural therapies if your child has experienced a physical trauma:

■ Give Bach Flower Rescue Remedy (also called Five Flowers Formula and Calming Essence) at the time of crisis and for at least one week following the event. Rescue Remedy will help ease any fear, panic, anxiety, or tension associated with the event.

■ To help alleviate any fear that persists after an emergency situation, try giving aspen or mimulus flower remedies. Aspen is indicated for a child with vague fears that she cannot explain or pinpoint. Mimulus is for the child with specific fears that she is able to identify.

■ Immediately following any trauma, give homeopathic *Arnica*. *Arnica* helps repair injured tissue and ease any physical and emotional shock associated with a traumatic event. Homeopathic *Hypericum* is useful if there has been an injury to nerves or to an area rich in nerve supply, such as the fingers, toes, tailbone, or head.

■ Immediately following an emergency in which the child is left afraid, restless, or anxious, give homeopathic *Aconite*, which has a calming effect.

■ American and Siberian Ginseng belong to a class of plants called adaptogens. They contain nutrients and trace minerals that will help strengthen the overall constitution if there is lingering fatigue.

■ Cover the basics with the following: lots of love and time spent together, a healthy whole foods diet, naps and plenty of nighttime sleep, appropriate exercise, and time spent outdoors. Each is an essential part of the healing process.

■ If necessary, you may want to consider counseling for your child. It is best to work with someone who specializes in working with children and who is trained in some sort of mind/body psychotherapy. The following organizations specialize in helping children and adults heal after a traumatic event:

Rocky Mountain
  Psychotherapy Associates
1777 Harrison Street, Suite 805
Denver, CO 80210
303–756–9989
Contact: Diane Heller
*This organization may be able
to refer you to a qualified
therapist in your area.*

Ergos Institute
  for Somatic Education
PO Box 110
Lyons, CO 80540
303–823–9524
Contact: Dr. Peter Levine
*This organization provides valuable
information on healing from
trauma.*

Natural Support Before and After Surgery

The following herbs, nutrients, and homeopathics are beneficial in helping to strengthen your child's body and prepare it for surgery, as well as speed the recovery time. If possible, begin giving your child the following items four to six weeks prior to the surgery. If the procedure is an emergency, begin giving them to your child once the surgery is over. Whatever the circumstances, continue giving these natural products to your child for six weeks after the procedure:

• B vitamins to promote wound healing.

• Vitamin C with bioflavonoids for their healing, anti-inflammatory, and immune-boosting properties.

• Zinc to help strengthen the immune system and promote wound healing.

• Echinacea and goldenseal to help boost the immune system and prevent infection.

• Gotu kola, taken orally, to enhance wound healing.

• Bromelain, an enzyme extracted from pineapple stems, for its natural anti-inflammatory properties. Give on an empty stomach.

Once the surgery is over, choose from the following natural products, which will further help in the healing process:

- Bach Flower Rescue Remedy (also called Five Flowers Formula and Calming Essence) to ease any fear, anxiety, tension, or emotional imbalance associated with the surgery.
- Homeopathic *Arnica* to help ease any fright.
- Acidophilus or bifidus to help your child maintain proper intestinal flora balance if he is taking antibiotics.
- Homeopathic *Nux vomica* to ease any nausea.
- Ginger tea or umeboshi paste to ease nausea.

Remember, although the surgery or other physical trauma may be over and the emergency has passed, your child still may need physical and emotional support (*see* Understanding Childhood Trauma After an Emergency beginning on page 19). Helping your child to completely rebuild and restore physical and emotional health is an invaluable gift.

Allergic Reactions

See ANAPHYLACTIC REACTION; FOOD ALLERGIES.

Anaphylactic Reaction

An anaphylactic reaction can be a severe and violent allergic response that may occur as a result of contact with an allergen. Possible allergens include chemicals, medicines, vaccines, particular foods or food additive—such as sulfites—and insect venom. An anaphylactic reaction may cause severe breathing distress and can be life threatening.

In anaphylaxis, the body's reaction to an allergen can cause a swelling of the air passages, with a consequent narrowing of the airway, resulting in extreme difficulty in breathing. In rare instances, your child's tongue and air passages may swell to the point where the airway closes and breathing becomes almost impossible.

Symptoms usually come on rapidly, most often within one to fifteen minutes of contact with an allergen. The more quickly a reaction begins, the more severe it is likely to be. The first signs that your child is suffering a reaction can include a sense of uneasiness, agitation, weakness, sweating, flushing, and shortness of breath, accompanied by intense fear and anxiety. Another early sign may be the presence of itchy hives that begin to spread rapidly all over the body. Other symptoms may include restlessness, falling blood pressure, shock, uneven heartbeat, wheezing, trouble swallowing, nausea, and diarrhea.

Seeing your child become terrified as she suffers this kind of an allergic reaction is frightening. But *don't panic*. As you seek treatment for your child, encourage her to calm down. Crying and screaming makes breathing even more difficult. If you become visibly upset, your child will only become more frightened. It is important that you remain calm and try to soothe her with reassuring words and your gentle touch.

EMERGENCY TREATMENT
FOR ANAPHYLACTIC REACTION

✚ At the slightest sign that your child may be having difficulty breathing due to a severe allergic reaction—especially if she has a history of such reactions—take her immediately to the emergency room of the nearest hospital. If you cannot transport your child yourself and must call for emergency help, stress the gravity of the situation. Seconds count. If an emergency adrenaline kit such as Ana-Guard, Ana-Kit, or EpiPen is available, administer it immediately. Follow this with 25 to 50 milligrams of diphen-hydranine (Benadryl) once. If Benadryl is not readily available, chlorpheniramine (Chlor-Trimeton or the equivalent) may be substituted. **Do not** give these medications to infants.

✚ **Do not** give your child anything to eat or drink while she is experiencing severe breathing distress.

CONVENTIONAL TREATMENT

■ Seek emergency medical help immediately. Emergency personnel may administer epinephrine (Adrenalin), an antihistamine (such as Benadryl), intravenous steroids (hydrocortisone or methyl prednisolone), or a bronchodilator (such as Alupent, Proventil, or Bronkosol) to counteract the allergen, decrease inflammation, and open the airway to restore free breathing. If treatment is begun soon enough, you can expect a dramatic easing of the situation. If your child's blood pressure is extremely low, intravenous fluids may be administered as well.

GENERAL RECOMMENDATIONS

■ If you know your child has a severe allergy, it is recommended that you have Ana-Guard or Ana-Kit on hand at home. These emergency adrenaline kits are easy to use and can be life saving.

■ After emergency treatment has been administered and the crisis is over, give your child Bach Flower Rescue Remedy—three drops, three times a day, for one week. Rescue Remedy will help to ease any fear, panic, anxiety, or tension.

■ In addition to Rescue Remedy, give your child one dose of homeopathic *Aconite* 30c as soon as possible after the crisis to help ease any fright.

Appendicitis

Appendicitis is an acute inflammation of the appendix, a thin, tube-shaped structure that protrudes from the first section of the large intestine. The appendix can become inflamed due either to an anatomical obstruction or a blockage of hardened feces. This inflammation can rapidly develop into an infection.

Symptoms of appendicitis usually begin with pain around the umbilicus that intensifies over several hours and moves to the lower right quadrant of the abdomen. This area will be very tender to even light pressure, and you may notice your child holding or protecting it. A decreased appetite, vomiting, and fever are frequently present. Diarrhea may be present as well, and extending the right leg may make the pain worse.

An inflamed appendix can burst, causing a life-threatening infection of the abdominal wall. If this happens, your child will rapidly become very ill, with a fever, pale color, and severe abdominal pain. Although a complaint of continuous abdominal pain is a key indicator of appendicitis, some children experience a milder onset of pain that comes and goes over several days before settling in as constant and severe. If you suspect appendicitis, seek immediate medical care.

SYMPTOMS OF APPENDICITIS

The main symptom of appendicitis is abdominal pain that is characterized by one or more of the following:

• It is localized on the right side of the abdomen, or it begins around the navel and gradually moves to the lower right quadrant of the abdomen.

• It is persistent, steady, and intensifies over a period of several hours.

• It feels worse if your child sneezes, coughs, or breathes deeply. It may feel worse if your child extends his right leg.

• The painful area is very tender to the touch.

• It is often accompanied by loss of appetite, nausea, vomiting, and fever.

If you suspect your child may be developing appendicitis, consult your doctor or seek emergency help immediately.

CONVENTIONAL TREATMENT

■ In order to diagnose appendicitis, a doctor will want to know details of when the pain began and the location and quality of the pain. Your doctor will do an abdominal and rectal exam, take a sample of blood to look for signs of an infection, and might order an x-ray or ultrasound scan to look for signs of blockage or inflammation.

■ If a diagnosis of appendicitis is confirmed, surgery to remove the inflamed appendix is the recommended course of treatment. Because of the danger that the appendix may rupture, surgery is usually done soon after the diagnosis is made.

■ To lower the risk of infection, your child may be given antibiotics before and immediately after surgery. If his appendix has ruptured, your child will definitely need intravenous antibiotics, and may need to be hospitalized for one to two weeks.

■ Because of the surgery and the manipulation of your child's digestive tract, the intestines will slow down, and may even stop moving for a day or two. Your child may have a nasogastric tube, a tube placed in the nose and down into the stomach, that uses suction to pull the contents of the stomach out of the body. This prevents nausea and vomiting. Except for an occasional ice chip, your child will not be able to eat or drink anything until his intestines begin working again. He will receive intravenous fluids to prevent dehydration and pain medication to help relieve discomfort.

■ Your child will have to get out of bed and walk the day after surgery. Even though this may seem like a daunting task, the importance of movement cannot be overemphasized. Among other things, walking helps the intestines to begin working again, and helps to prevent pneumonia from developing.

GENERAL RECOMMENDATIONS

■ To ensure a full and strong recovery after surgery, adequate rest is essential. Limit visitors and create a calm and familiar environment.

■ Once discharged from the hospital, your child will have periods of fatigue. Resuming a daily routine is probably fine, although he may need more rest than usual until his full strength is back.

■ Contact sports, heavy lifting, and abdominal exercises must be avoided for as long as your doctor recommends, probably for six to eight weeks after surgery.

■ Follow the post surgery and wound healing recommendations for natural support before and after surgery described on page 61.

■ Give your child either an acidophilus or bifidus supplement to help restore the healthy flora of the large intestines.

Asthma

Asthma is an inflammatory respiratory illness characterized by mild to severe difficulty in breathing. This is caused by constriction and swelling of the airways, and an increase in mucus secretions, which plug up the smaller passages. As a result, air cannot get into or out of the lungs easily. Wheezing results as air squeaks through the narrowed, inflamed passages. An asthma attack can cause such shortness of breath and poor oxygen intake that a child may need to be hospitalized.

Asthma can be triggered by a variety of things, including pollen, dust, feathers, molds, animal dander, pollution, cigarette smoke, or cold dry air, as well as an upper respiratory infection, exercise, excitement, and stress. A child can develop an asthma attack for no apparent reason.

A child experiencing an asthma attack will cough, wheeze, have an increased respiratory rate, have a feeling of tightness in her chest, and have difficulty breathing. Early signs include an itchy throat, a change in breathing pattern, fatigue, paleness, nervousness, a runny nose, or moodiness. It is important to watch your child carefully and treat her quickly if you notice an asthma attack coming on. If you have any doubts as to your child's breathing, don't hesitate to call your doctor.

If your child suffers from asthma, one simple way you can monitor her breathing is with an instrument called a *peak flow meter*, available at many large drugstores. This also can be ordered through medical supply catalogs. It is a relatively inexpensive, simple-to-use device that measures how much air pressure your child can exert with a full exhalation. The meter's indicator can be used to compare how your child's air flow changes from day to day. By monitoring this way, you will have a more reliable means of determining whether your child's condition is getting better or worse. Your physician will help you determine what to watch for with your child.

EMERGENCY TREATMENT
FOR ASTHMA

✚ In the event of a severe asthma attack, you need to seek immediate medical care for your child. If your child's asthma is not resolving using the treatments you know, call your physician and take your child to the nearest emergency room.

✚ At the hospital, your child will probably be given an inhaled medication that sprays a bronchodilator (a substance that opens air passages to restore free breathing) directly into the airways. If this does not help, she may receive other drugs, such as intravenous steroids or theophylline, and may need to be hospitalized. In some cases, a child will need to receive oxygen to ease the work of breathing.

CONVENTIONAL TREATMENT

■ For chronic asthma, steroids are currently the conventional treatment of choice. These medicines work by decreasing the swelling and inflammation of the airways. They can be taken orally or inhaled. Inhaled steroids (including Beclovent, Vanceril, AeroBid, and Azmacort) are more commonly used; oral steroids (such as Pediapred) are generally used only in more severe cases. All steroids potentially have significant side effects, especially when taken over the long term, that need to be understood. Talk this over with your doctor or nurse.

■ Bronchodilators, in either oral or inhaled form, may be prescribed for the relief of occasional symptoms of asthma. These medications work to open up the airways, easing breathing. Inhaled bronchodilators that may be prescribed include Alupent, Maxair, Proventil, and Ventolin. Oral medications in this category (which include Alupent and theophylline-based drugs) are rarely used today because they can cause side effects such as restlessness, insomnia, headache, loss of appetite, increased heart rate, dizziness, nausea, and vomiting. Long-term use of theophylline may also be associated with behavioral problems and learning disabilities, although the evidence for this is not conclusive.

GENERAL RECOMMENDATIONS

■ Once the crisis of an asthma attack is over, give your child Bach Flower Rescue Remedy—three drops, three times a day, for a week. If your child is able to drink during the attack, it can be helpful to give Rescue Remedy during this time as well. Rescue Remedy will help to ease any fear, panic, anxiety, or tension.

■ After the emergency, give your child licorice root tea—one cup, three times a day, for three days. This tea will help calm and soothe the respiratory tract.

Caution: Do not give licorice to a child with high blood pressure.

■ Proper nutrition, homeopathic and herbal treatments, and acupressure can be helpful in preventing further asthma attacks.

Back Injury

See BONES, BROKEN.

Bites, Animal and Human

See also BITES, SNAKE; BITES AND STINGS, INSECT.

Should your child suffer a bite that breaks the skin, prompt medical care is essential. This applies whether the bite is from a playmate, a wild or stray animal, or the family pet.

EMERGENCY TREATMENT
FOR ANIMAL AND HUMAN BITES

✚ If your child suffers a bite that breaks the skin, immediately and thoroughly disinfect the area with lots of water, soap, and hydrogen peroxide. Bite wounds that break the skin can easily become infected. This is true of human as well as animal bites. Human saliva is often alive with infectious bacteria.

✚ If your child has been bitten by an animal, try to confine the animal so it can be tested for rabies. If the animal belongs to a neighbor, be sure you can identify the owner. If you can determine that the animal is not rabid, your child can be spared the very uncomfortable (but otherwise necessary) treatment with rabies vaccine. If the animal is wild and you cannot capture it, your child will have to be treated for rabies.

✚ Call your physician or take your child to the emergency room, or call for emergency help. Any child who receives a bite wound that breaks the skin should be examined and treated by a doctor.

CONVENTIONAL TREATMENT

■ Your child's bite wound will be cleansed, treated with a topical antibiotic such as Betadine or a triple-antibiotic ointment such as bacitracin or neomycin, and bandaged. You will probably be instructed to change the dressing daily with a new application of antibiotic at each change. If necessary, the wound will be stitched closed. If the wound is very deep, involves the hands or knuckles, or involves damage to tendons that requires repair, surgery may be recommended to thoroughly clean the affected tissues and close the wound before bandaging.

■ After emergency first aid has been administered, your child will be given an injection to update her immunity to tetanus if necessary. If your child was bitten by an animal and it cannot be determined that the animal is *not* infected with rabies, rabies immune globulin will be administered. A bite from a rabid animal can be fatal unless the victim receives immediate medical treatment, which consists of a series of injections into the muscles over a period of twenty-eight days and again at ninety days.

■ Once the wound is thoroughly cleansed and bandaged, and any necessary immunizations have been given, an oral antibiotic such as ampicillin, cephalexin (Keflex), clindamycin, or dicloxacillin may be prescribed to prevent infection.

■ Until it heals, your child's wound will need to be checked every few days for signs of infection and treated accordingly.

GENERAL RECOMMENDATIONS

■ Once the wound has been treated, give your child the homeopathic *Ledum* 12c or 12x, three times a day, for three days. *Ledum* is helpful for easing pain and healing any bite or puncture wound.

■ After emergency treatment has been administered, give your child echinacea and goldenseal. These herbals will help resolve or prevent infection.

Bites, Snake

There are many varieties of poisonous snakes. Because a child's small body has less of a capacity for fighting a reaction to snake venom, prompt medical care for snakebite is essential.

Symptoms caused by snakebite range from mild to severe, and can include a racing pulse with swelling and discoloration around the area of the bite. If your child is bitten by a snake, he may feel weak and be short of breath; he will probably feel nauseous and may vomit. If the venom is very strong, your child will experience severe pain and much swelling. His pupils will dilate, and shock and convulsion may occur. Your child may twitch uncontrollably and his speech may become slurred. After a severe snakebite, a child can become paralyzed and lose consciousness. If your child is bitten by a snake, act fast.

EMERGENCY TREATMENT
FOR SNAKEBITE

✚ Take your child immediately to the emergency room of the nearest hospital, or call emergency medical personnel. ***Medical intervention is essential.***

✚ If medical care is not immediately available, stay calm. Reassure your child, speaking calmly to prevent panic, and follow these steps:

1. Have your child lie down and rest quietly. Activity can spread the venom throughout the body.

2. Immobilize the affected limb. If possible, keep it at the same level as the heart.

3. If a venom extractor is available, apply suction immediately. It takes at least three minutes to begin adequate poison extraction. Continue suctioning out the venom for at least fifteen minutes, or until you can secure medical care for your child.

4. *Do not* make an incision into the bite or suck the poison out with your mouth. Both actions create more problems than they solve.

5. *Do not* use an ice pack on the wound. Cold therapy is not recommended for snake bites, as it can damage tissues.

6. Call your local Poison Control Center for instructions on how best to treat your child (*see* listings beginning on page 155).

7. Seek medical care as soon as possible.

CONVENTIONAL TREATMENT

■ Seek emergency treatment. Rely on medical personnel to take the appropriate measures. The primary treatment for snakebite is the use of intravenous antivenin. It is important to go to a hospital that is experienced in its use.

■ Once the wound has been treated and your child has recovered sufficiently from the effects of the injury to leave the hospital, medical personnel will advise you on the proper way to care for him as he recovers.

GENERAL RECOMMENDATIONS

■ Make sure you know how to identify all types of venomous snakes that are indigenous to your area. Should a medical emergency arise, knowing the species of the snake that attacked your child will save precious time.

■ Along with your usual first aid supplies, keep a snakebite kit readily available, especially when camping out. We recommend The Extractor from Sawyer Products, which is available in many camping and outdoor equipment stores or directly from the company. They can be contacted at P.O. Box 188, Safety Harbor, FL 34695; telephone 813–725–1177.

■ After emergency treatment has been given, to further help your child recover from a snakebite, give homeopathic *Lachesis* 12x or 6c, three times a day on day one; give *Ledum* 12x or 12c, three times a day on day two; and give *Staphysagria* 30x or 30c, three times a day on day three.

■ Once the wound has been treated, give your child an echinacea and goldenseal combination to help prevent infection and to clear the toxin from the body. Treating snakebites was one of the original uses for echinacea.

PREVENTION

■ Most snakebites occur on unprotected ankles and legs. Shorts and sneakers don't provide adequate protection. Outfit your child with tough hiking boots and suitable pants, such as heavy jeans, for tramping through the woods or going on a hiking trip.

■ Teach your child not to poke sticks into inviting holes or stick his hands into underbrush.

■ When camping out, don't permit your child to go exploring alone.

Bites and Stings, Insect

Bites and stings from most common insects, such as mosquitoes, gnats, fleas, common spiders, ants, and other "creepy crawlies" can cause itchy welts on arms and legs. A bee, wasp, or hornet sting can cause swelling and stinging at the site. Usually, bites and stings are no more than an annoyance and cause only slight local swelling and irritation.

There are exceptions, however, such as a bite from a venomous insect like the brown recluse or black widow spider, or a severe allergic reaction to a bee sting. A bite from a tiny deer tick may cause a large circular lesion that progresses into a rash of small round lesions. The deer tick is the insect responsible for transmitting Lyme disease, and the characteristic bull's-eye rash is often the first sign of that illness.

If your child is stung by a bee, wasp, or hornet, or bitten by an insect you suspect may be poisonous (such as the black widow or brown recluse spider), she may need emergency medical treatment.

EMERGENCY TREATMENT
FOR INSECT BITES AND STINGS

✚ **For venomous spider bites, get immediate help.** If you suspect that your child has been bitten by a venomous insect, such as the black widow or brown recluse spider, take her immediately to the emergency room of the nearest hospital. If you cannot transport your child, call for emergency help and explain the situation. In the very beginning stages, the only way you will know that a child has been bitten by a poisonous spider is if you see the spider in the vicinity. If possible, capture the insect and have it ready to show the doctor for quick identification.

If your child is bitten by an insect or spider you can't identify, call your local Poison Control Center for instructions on how best to treat your child (see page 155 for a complete listing of Poison Control Centers).

✚ **For black widow spider bites.** The poisonous venom of the black widow spider causes sweating, stomach cramps, nausea, headaches, and dizziness. A small child bitten by a black widow is especially endangered. Treatment for a black widow bite consists of the injection of antivenin. The antivenin itself, however, can cause an allergic reaction in some people. A known allergy to this drug or to horse serum prohibits its use. After administering the antivenin, medical personnel will monitor your child. They may also give your child muscle relaxants or intravenous calcium to relieve muscle pain and spasms.

✚ **For brown recluse spider bites.** A bite from the poisonous brown recluse spider will cause a rapidly expanding red blister surrounded by white and red circles. Pain, nausea, fever, and chills are common. Because a small child can have a serious reaction to this venom, medical care is essential. If the bite is untreated, a large amount of the surrounding tissue can die, requiring surgical excision. Brown recluse spider bites may be treated with injections of steroids. A drug called Dapsone is also effective in some cases.

✚ **For bee, wasp, or hornet stings.** Should your child be stung by a bee, wasp, or hornet, remove the stinger by gently scraping it out, then wash and rinse the area thoroughly. Watch your child carefully for signs of an allergic reaction, such as redness that begins spreading rapidly outward from the area of penetration, hives, or difficulty breathing. Reactions can occur within minutes or after several hours, so keep a watchful eye on your child.

At the first sign of a severe allergic reaction, especially if your child is having difficulty breathing, take her to the emergency room of the nearest hospital. If you cannot transport your child, call for emergency help and stress the gravity of the situation. Seconds count. If an emergency adrenaline kit such as Ana-Guard, Ana-Kit, or EpiPen is available, administer it immediately. These kits, which are available by prescription only, contain a syringe filled with a premeasured dose of epinephrine, a hormone that opens the airways and restores free breathing to combat a life-threatening allergic reaction.

✚ **For tick bites.** Although many tick bites are harmless, if your child has been bitten by a tick, it is wise to have the tick—and your child—tested for infection. The deer tick, most prevalent in the northeastern United States, is responsible for the transmission of Lyme disease—a potentially serious long-term illness.

First, remove the tick carefully by grabbing it with a tweezers at the point of contact and pulling it off firmly. Do not twist or squeeze the tick, as this can cause bacteria to be released. A slow, steady pull is recommended. Place the tick in a sealed container with a blade of grass or a moistened cotton ball. Cleanse the site of the bite with alcohol, and apply an antibiotic ointment. Then take your child and the tick to the doctor. Blood tests for Lyme disease are available, and your doctor may prescribe a precautionary course of treatment as well.

The first sign noted in most people with Lyme disease is a characteristic "bull's-eye" marking at the site of the tick bite. This is a round, raised reddish lesion that typically is paler, even white, in the center. In some cases, the bull's-eye rash gradually expands in the center; in others, a bumpy rash develops on the torso. These signs may come and go throughout the course of the disease. Often accompanying the development of the bull's-eye mark and/or rash are flulike symptoms, including fever, chills, headache, and overall achiness. Some people develop an enlarged spleen and lymph glands, some complain of sore throat and severe headache, and some suffer from nausea and vomiting. The symptoms can occur singly or in combination, and they can develop anywhere from three days to three weeks after the initial bite.

The critical factor in the treatment of Lyme disease is early diagnosis. If you suspect that your child may be developing Lyme disease, consult your doctor.

✚ **For common insect bites.** Monitor your child's reactions. If she should suffer a serious allergic or toxic reaction after a bite or sting from a common insect, take her to the emergency room of the nearest hospital. If your child seems listless or unlike her normal self following a bite or sting, call your physician immediately.

GENERAL RECOMMENDATIONS

■ If your child has a severe allergy to bites or stings, make sure she wears a Medic Alert bracelet. The information the bracelet carries will alert those around your child to her needs in the event of an allergic reaction. Contact Medic Alert at 2323 Colorado Avenue, Turlock, CA 95380; telephone 800–432–5378.

■ If your child is stung by a bee and you know she is allergic to bee venom, seek immediate medical care. Should your child develop respiratory symptoms, such as wheezing or difficulty breathing, take her to the emergency room of the nearest hospital. A child rarely has a problem with her first bee sting. However, if there is a family history of allergies, or if your child exhibits a strong reaction to her first bee sting, a life-threatening allergy may develop.

■ If you know that your child could suffer a severe allergic reaction to a bite or sting, ask your doctor about the possibility of prescribing emergency medication for quick administration. Epinephrine, which can open your child's airways and restore free breathing in a crisis, is available for home use as the Ana-Kit or EpiPen, which contains a syringe with a premeasured dose of medication.

■ If your child is stung by a bee, wasp, or hornet, remove the stinger by gently scraping it out, not by pulling. Watch your child closely for any allergic reaction.

■ If your child is prone to stings, it may be worthwhile to invest in The Extractor, a device that can be used to extract venom from a bite or sting. It is available in many camping and outdoor equipment stores or directly through the manufacturer, Sawyer Products. Their address is P.O. Box 188, Safety Harbor, FL 34695; telephone 813–725–1177.

■ Treat minor insect bites, stings, and itches with a cold compress or ice to help stop the spread of histamine, the chemical that causes itching.

■ Sweating increases the discomfort of most skin irritations. Try to keep your child's skin cool and dry.

■ Compresses of salt water or lemon juice can help lessen the itching or pain of an insect bite or sting.

■ Once the wound has been treated, give your child the homeopathic *Apis* 6c or 12x, three times a day, for three days. *Apis* is helpful in the treatment of large, red, swollen insect bites.

■ The homeopathic *Urtica urens* is effective in alleviating the itchiness of insect bites or stings. After the wound has been treated, give your child *Urtica urens* 6c or 12x, three times a day, for three days. Topical *Urtica urens* ointment or gel is also effective.

PREVENTION

■ There are many commercial insect repellents sold over the counter. These formulas may not be safe for children, however. The chemical ingredients they contain can be absorbed through the skin in doses that may be toxic to youngsters, causing headaches and other problems.

■ Citronella is a safe, natural repellent that may be applied to your child's exposed skin. Oil of citronella is usually available in health food stores. Natrapel is a typical citronella product.

Caution: Some children are allergic to citronella.

■ Deet (diethyl toluamide) is a very effective insect repellent, but because of its high potential toxicity, it is not usually recommended for children. However, a very low dose formulation of deet is available that is safer for children. It is called Skedaddle! and is produced by Little Point Corporation of Cambridge, Massachusetts. One application of this repellent lasts for four to six hours.

■ Garlic helps to repel insects. Give your child one or two capsules, twice daily, for three days before a wilderness outing and throughout the trip.

■ Spray permethrin (available as Nix, Permanone, or Duranon) on your child's clothes. This is a medication normally used to get rid of head lice. It is very effective and virtually nontoxic when used this way as an insect repellent. One spraying can last for up to two weeks. Permethrin binds strongly to cellulose, which is the main component of most clothing.

■ Liquid vitamin B, taken orally, is effective in preventing some insect bites. Vitamin B is excreted through the skin and is believed to leave a bad taste in the mouths of mosquitoes and fleas. Before a trip to the woods, give your child 1 teaspoon of liquid vitamin-B complex, twice daily, for three days, and continue giving it throughout the trip.

■ Teach your child not to chase bees, wasps, or hornets. If you spot a nest built by one of these stinging insects, warn your child to stay well away.

■ Don't swat at or squash a yellow jacket. Recent studies show that the body of a crushed yellow jacket exudes a chemical that attracts and stimulates other yellow jackets in the area to attack. If you're being bothered by a yellow jacket, it's better to leave the area.

■ Cologne, shiny jewelry, and even perfumed suntan lotions all attract insects. It's best not to use or wear them when spending time outdoors.

Black Eye

See EYE INJURIES.

Bleeding, Internal

If your child has been involved in an accident and has broken a bone, ruptured an internal organ, or suffered a blow to the abdomen or head, internal bleeding may result. Internal bleeding occurs when blood leaks from damaged vessels inside the body into body cavities, such as the abdomen, chest, or skull, or into other tissues.

Internal bleeding is not easily observed from outside. Signs of internal bleeding can include a rigid, tight abdomen; a tight, painful chest; blood in the vomit or stool; or a trickle of blood coming from the mouth, nose, or ear. Bright red, frothy blood tends to be coming from the lungs; dark red or black blood tends to be coming from the stomach. Internal bleeding can cause your child to go into shock.

A definitive diagnosis of internal bleeding must usually be made by a physician, who will rely on x-rays, laboratory tests, and blood measurements to assess your child's condition.

EMERGENCY TREATMENT FOR INTERNAL BLEEDING

✚ If you suspect that your child may be bleeding internally, call for emergency help and stress the urgency of the situation. As you wait for help to arrive, have your child lie down in one of the following manners:

- If your child is conscious and not vomiting, place her on her back with a small pillow under her head, which should be turned to one side.

- If your child is unconscious, place her on her side. If she begins vomiting, this position will help prevent her from inhaling material into her lungs.

✚ Cover your child lightly with a blanket and keep her still. Do not give her anything by mouth—no medicine or food, or liquid of any kind—before a doctor has assessed the situation, and do not move her. Stay with your child, and try to remain calm and reassuring. Rely on medical personnel to take the appropriate emergency steps to stabilize your child's condition and prepare her body for transport to the hospital.

CONVENTIONAL TREATMENT

■ Be prepared for the possibility that your child may require a blood transfusion or the administration of intravenous saline solution to maintain fluid levels even before reaching the hospital. Upon arrival at the hospital, a child with internal bleeding will likely need immediate surgery to repair the damage that is causing the bleeding.

■ After surgery, your child may be put in an intensive care unit and monitored closely until her condition has stabilized and she can begin the process of recovery.

GENERAL RECOMMENDATIONS

■ Once the crisis is over and emergency treatment has been administered, give your child American or Siberian ginseng—one dose, twice a day, for one month. These herbs will help nourish and strengthen the system and resolve any lingering fatigue or weakness.

■ After the emergency, you may want to talk to your doctor about giving your child a B12 injection. This treatment will enhance the body's ability to produce red blood cells. Liquid B12 vitamins are also helpful if you do not want to give your child an injection.

Bleeding, Nose

See NOSEBLEED.

Bleeding, Severe (Hemorrhage)

See also BLEEDING, INTERNAL; CUTS AND SCRAPES; NOSEBLEED.

All healthy, active children get cuts and scrapes from time to time, and for the most part these minor injuries can be treated at home. But if your child receives a severe external wound that spurts blood or causes a great deal of steady bleeding, it is possible that an artery or vein has been cut. Arteries carry oxygen-rich blood from the lungs and heart to the rest of the body; veins carry oxygen-poor blood back to the heart and lungs. If an artery is cut, it will bleed oxygenated blood that is bright red in color. Oxygen-poor blood coming from a cut vein is a dark, bluish red.

The body of a toddler who weighs twenty-five pounds contains only about one quart of blood. An older child has from three to six quarts of blood, depending on body size. Hundreds of miles of blood vessels run throughout the body to every living organ and tissue (except for the cornea of the eye). If blood flow to any part of the body is cut off, that part will die. Brain cells die after three to four minutes without a fresh supply of blood.

EMERGENCY TREATMENT FOR SEVERE BLEEDING

✚ Have someone call immediately for emergency help.

✚ Cover the bleeding wound with a clean cloth or gauze, and quickly apply very firm, steady pressure. If there is no clean cloth or gauze immediately available, use your bare hand to apply pressure. Even if your child complains that the pressure hurts, continue applying very firm, steady pressure. It is necessary to stop the bleeding. If the wound has a foreign object, such as a piece of glass or wood, be careful not to push it further into the wound with your pressure.

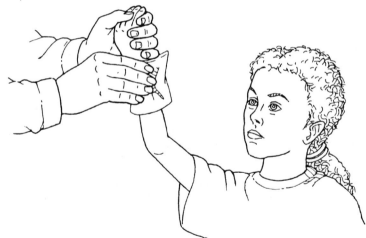

✚ If there is no suspicion of a spinal injury, raise the wound above the level of the heart to help minimize the amount of blood that spurts from the wound with every heartbeat (see above). Signs of a spinal injury include pain at the site of the injury, weakness or numbness in an extremity, inability to move an extremity, or lack of feeling in an extremity. If any of these signs are present, **do not** move your child. If you do, you may worsen the injury.

✚ If the blood soaks through the cloth pad or gauze, put more cloth or gauze over the old pad and continue applying pressure. Do not remove the original blood-soaked pad. Early clotting may become dislodged.

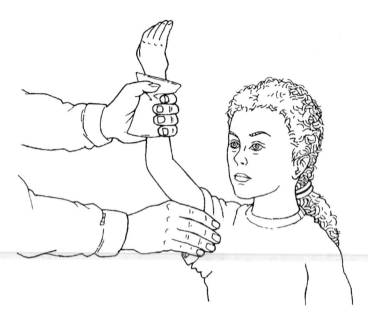

✚ If steady pressure and elevation cannot control the bleeding, place additional pressure with your fingers and thumb on the pressure point that is closest to the injury and between the injury and the heart (*see* above). If the femoral artery, located in the groin area, is to be compressed, use the heel of your hand. (*See* page 83 for location of pressure points.)

✚ If emergency medical personnel are not on their way to you, take your child to the emergency room of the nearest hospital. If you are fortunate enough to have another adult with you, have that person see to the transportation while you hold your child and continue applying pressure. If you are alone with your child and must drive him yourself, tie cloth or gauze very firmly in place to maintain pressure on the wound. If you must tie on a bandage, check for a pulse beat below it to make sure the tissues are receiving an adequate supply of blood.

✚ A tourniquet is a bandage that is tied so tightly that it cuts off the flow of blood to an area of the body, usually a portion of an arm or leg. It is a drastic measure that is appropriate only if blood loss is so severe and rapid as to be immediately life threatening. ***Do not apply a tourniquet unless it is absolutely necessary and then only as a last resort.*** Because it cuts off blood, a tourniquet deprives the tissues below the wound of oxygen, creating the risk of your child losing a limb. If your child is losing so much blood so rapidly that you must put on a tourniquet, be sure to mark it with the time the tourniquet was applied. Never cover a tourniquet. It is vital that medical personnel can see immediately that a tourniquet is in place.

✚ A severe loss of blood will cause shock, which can be life threatening. Try to remain calm and reassuring. Any panic you display will be transmitted to your child and make the situation worse. Your immediate task is to stem the flow of blood and secure emergency medical care for your child.

✚ Do not give your child any medicine or food, or liquid of any kind, before a doctor has assessed the situation. It is important that your child's stomach be empty, as surgery may be needed to repair the wound.

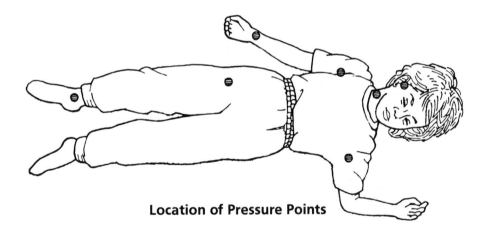

Location of Pressure Points

CONVENTIONAL TREATMENT

■ Seek emergency medical treatment (beginning on page 81). Rely on medical personnel to take over and do what is necessary and appropriate to stop the bleeding and stabilize your child's body. He may require a blood transfusion or the administration of intravenous saline solution to maintain fluid levels.

■ On reaching the hospital, your child may require sutures (stitches) or surgery to repair the damage that caused the bleeding.

■ Once the wound has been treated and your child is well enough to leave the hospital, medical personnel will advise you on the proper way to care for your child as he recovers from his injury. Ask your doctor for recommendations regarding diet, activity level, special exercises, and any measures necessary to guard against complications.

GENERAL RECOMMENDATIONS

■ Once the crisis is over and emergency treatment has been administered, give your child American or Siberian ginseng—one dose, twice a day, for one month. These herbs will help nourish and strengthen the system and resolve any lingering fatigue or weakness.

■ After the emergency, you may want to talk to your doctor about giving your child a B12 injection. This treatment will enhance the body's ability to produce red blood cells. Liquid B12 vitamins are also helpful if you do not want to give your child an injection.

Bones, Broken (Fractures)

When people think of bones, they often visualize them as "dead," rather like the dry skeletons that sometimes hang in science classrooms. But bones are really living tissue with a rich supply of blood vessels and nerves. As a result, a bone fracture is not only painful, it causes shock and trauma to the whole body.

Because a child's bones are still growing, correct treatment of a broken bone is especially important in childhood. If not treated correctly, a child may lose mobility and partial function of the bone.

If your child has suffered an accident, a bad fall, or a hard blow, he may have broken a bone. Depending on the cause of the break, there may be an open wound near the fracture. Your child may lie very still to protect himself against the pain of movement. An affected limb may appear crooked or bent. The area near a fracture will be painful or tender when moved or touched, and may appear swollen, red, and bruised.

Depending on which bone is broken, there is a possibility of additional damage, including internal bleeding. A broken rib may puncture a lung;

a broken vertebra can damage the spinal cord; a skull fracture can cause bleeding into the skull. Broken bones should be taken seriously and treated immediately.

EMERGENCY TREATMENT FOR BROKEN BONES

✚ If you think your child may have suffered a serious bone fracture—a broken long bone, rib, or vertebra, or a skull fractures or a neck or back injury, **do not move him.** Movement can cause additional injury. Call for emergency help.

✚ Remain calm and reassure your child. Your soothing presence, familiar voice, and gentle touch may be the most helpful things you can offer to your child.

✚ If you have taken a first aid course and are very confident of your ability, you can use a splint to immobilize a broken limb, including the joints above and below the fracture. This is a temporary measure, of course. A doctor's evaluation and treatment are still essential. (See emergency guidelines for Immobilizing a Broken Bone, beginning on page 40, and Immobilizing an Injured Head, Neck, and Back on page 44.)

✚ If your child has broken a small bone such as a finger or toe, apply ice or a cool compress to the injury and elevate it above the level of the heart. This will minimize swelling and help relieve pain. Take your child to the nearest emergency room or to your physician.

✚ Noses are seldom actually broken. A child's nose is made of cartilage, not bone. A blow to the nose can be very painful, however. A blood-filled bruise may develop inside the nose, causing a black eye on one or both sides. Apply an ice pack immediately. With the ice in place, take your child to the emergency room or to your physician for prompt attention.

CONVENTIONAL TREATMENT

■ On arrival at the hospital, your child will be examined. A broken bone must be assessed, x-rayed, set, and possibly placed in traction by a physician.

■ The possibility of internal damage will be considered. Should any further injury come to light, emergency room personnel will take the appropriate measures.

■ If your child is in pain, pain medication may be administered.

■ The proper setting and casting of the long bones of the arms and legs are particularly critical in a still-growing child. The doctor must take care to ensure that these bones continue to grow steadily and match the growth of their counterparts.

■ Broken fingers and toes may be splinted, or the doctor may securely tape the injured digit to adjacent fingers or toes. Either method will keep the bone immobilized while it heals.

GENERAL RECOMMENDATIONS

■ A SAM splint is an emergency splint made of foam-lined laminated aluminum. Available in most pharmacies, a SAM splint is a good item to have in your home health kit.

■ To help the broken bone heal, it is important to supplement your child's diet with certain nutrients. These nutrients include calcium, magnesium, vitamin D, zinc, and trace minerals.

■ Once the emergency is over and proper medical attention has been given, a number of homeopathic remedies will further help heal the traumatized tissue and broken bone. After the bone has been set, give your child *Arnica* 30c, three times a day, for three days. Then give her *Symphytum* 12c, three times a day, for three days. Finally, give your child *Calcarea phosphorica* 6c or 12x, three times a day, for one week.

Breathing Distress

See ANAPHYLACTIC REACTION; ASTHMA; UNCONSCIOUSNESS.

Bruises

When your child develops a bruise, a "black-and-blue mark," or a black eye, it is because an injury to a blood vessel has caused blood to leak into the surrounding tissue. Bruises are usually caused by an injury to the small capillaries located near the surface of the skin. These tiny blood vessels heal fairly quickly. As the body reabsorbs the blood, the characteristic mark disappears.

Because there are many blood vessels in the head, when a child falls and hits her head, there can be a lot of bleeding into surrounding tissue, causing the classic "goose egg." A blow to the forehead or nose can cause blood to accumulate in the surrounding loose tissues, resulting in the condition commonly known as a black eye.

A new bruise will be tender to the touch and may be swollen. A bruise generally starts out as a red mark, then turns the classic black-and-blue or purple color. As the bruise fades, it becomes lighter and sometimes a bit yellow or brown from residual iron that is left over after the blood fluids are reabsorbed.

EMERGENCY TREATMENT FOR BRUISES

✚ Immediately after an injury, elevate the affected area.

✚ Put ice on the bruise for five to ten minutes (if you can persuade your child to sit still long enough), then take the ice off for forty-five minutes. Repeat this cycle at least three to five times immediately following the injury, and as much as possible for the first day or two afterward. To avoid causing frostbite damage to the tissues, place a towel or washcloth between the ice and the skin, and be careful not to leave the ice in place too long.

GENERAL RECOMMENDATIONS

■ Apply ice or a cold compress to the area, as described above.

■ If your child suffers a blow that results in a black eye, be alert for any signs that her vision has been affected. If you suspect any vision impairment, consult an ophthalmologist. (For information on treating black eyes, *see* EYE INJURIES.)

■ After proper emergency treatment has been administered, apply homeopathic *Arnica* gel or ointment if the skin is not broken. Give your child *Arnica* 30c internally, three times a day, for two days.

■ Bromelain, an enzyme extracted from pineapple stems, is a natural anti-inflammatory and can help resolve the bruise.

■ Bioflavonoids can help heal small blood vessels.

Burns

See also SUNBURN.

Your child may suffer a burn from dry heat (fire or sun); moist heat (steam or hot liquids); corrosive chemicals; or electricity.

An encounter with electricity can be particularly dangerous. A severe electrical shock may knock your child unconscious, and he may stop breathing. There may be deep burns at the point where the current entered and exited the body, as well as internal damage.

Depending on the location, extent, and cause of the burn, your child may need immediate medical care. A burn can cause scarring, which may limit functioning of the burned area. Regardless of their size and severity, burns on the face, the palms of the hands, the soles of the feet, and on or near a joint can have serious implications. Burns in these areas should always be checked by a doctor and watched with special care. Any burn should be watched for signs of a possible infection.

When evaluating your child's burn, here's what to look for:

• A *first-degree burn* involves only the epidermis, the upper layer of the skin. The area is hot, red, and painful, but without swelling or blistering. Sunburn is usually a first-degree burn.

• A *second-degree burn* involves the epidermis and part of the underlying skin layers. The pain is severe. The area is pink or red and mottled, and is usually moist and seeping, moderately swollen, and blistered.

Fire Safety for Children

A child who knows basic fire safety rules is less likely to suffer needless injury. As soon as your child is old enough to understand, teach him to do the following in the event of a fire:

- Shout "Fire!" to alert others.

- Leave the building immediately. **Do not** stop to pick up anything. **Do not** try to put out the fire.

- As you leave the building, feel each door before opening it. If a door is hot, find another way out. Always close doors behind you as you leave.

- Crouch close to the floor, or crawl if necessary. There is less smoke lower down. Cover your face with a cloth (a damp one is best) and breathe shallowly through the fabric.

- As soon as you escape the building, summon help. Go to a neighbor's or dial 911 or 0 from a nearby telephone and ask for emergency assistance.

- If your clothes catch on fire, immediately stop moving, drop to the ground, and roll over to extinguish the flames, all the while shouting "Fire!"

Practice these techniques with your child so that he will know what to do if fire should strike.

- Because it involves injury to all layers of the skin, a *third-degree burn* is also called a *full-thickness burn*. This severe burn destroys the nerves and blood vessels in the skin. Because the nerves are damaged, there is little or no pain at first. The affected area may be white, yellow, black, or cherry red. The skin may appear dry and leathery.

- A *fourth-degree burn* extends through the skin and penetrates into underlying structures, such as muscle and bone. It looks and feels like a third-degree burn, but it does greater damage to the body.

EMERGENCY TREATMENT FOR BURNS

✚ **Remove the cause.** All burns should be treated first by removing the cause—putting out flames, washing off chemicals, or breaking electrical contact. If your child's clothing is on fire, douse him with water or wrap him in a blanket and place him on the ground to put out the flames.

✚ **For electrical burns.** In the case of electrical shock, your inclination will probably be to snatch your child out of harm's way. ***Don't.*** You may receive a severe shock yourself and become unable to help your child. To break electrical contact safely, first switch off the current. If that is not possible (as in the case of a live wire) use a nonconductive item, such as a wooden broom handle, to lift or push the source of the current away from your child. Always take your child to the emergency room for medical evaluation after an electrical burn, even if he seems to have suffered only a minor burn.

✚ **For chemical burns.** If your child suffers a chemical burn from a corrosive liquid, immediately flood the area with cool running water to dilute and wash away the chemical.

✚ **Assess your child's condition.** Once the cause of the burn has been removed, check your child's breathing and pulse. *If your child's breathing or pulse has stopped, turn to* CARDIOPULMONARY RESUSCITATION (CPR) *on page 33. Start CPR at once.* Have someone call for emergency help.

✚ **For third- or fourth-degree burns.** If the burn is deep and severe, your child will require immediate medical attention. Do not remove any clothing that is stuck to the burn, but lightly cover the area with a clean white cloth. Call for emergency medical assistance or take your child immediately to the emergency room of the nearest hospital. Do not attempt to treat a severe third- or fourth-degree burn at home.

✚ **For first- or second-degree burns.** To minimize damage from a first- or second-degree burn, cool the burn as rapidly as possible. Immerse the affected area in cool running water until the stinging and burning sensations lessen. This may take ten minutes or even longer. Do not stop prematurely.

If the burn occurs through clothing (as in a spill of hot liquid), don't wait to strip the clothes from your child. Immediately immerse the area in cool, running water. Remove the wet clothes from your child while cooling the burn. Also, remove any watches, bracelets, rings, belts, or other constricting items from the area before the burn swells.

✚ **For burns in sensitive areas.** The thin, tender skin of a child is particularly susceptible to burns. Take your child to the emergency room if a burn appears severe or extensive, or if the burned area is on the face, the palms of the hands, the soles of the feet, or on or near a joint.

✚ **Avoid worsening the injury.** *Do not* apply butter, oil, grease, lotions, or creams to burns. *Do not* cover burns with adhesive dressings or fluffy materials.

CONVENTIONAL TREATMENT

■ A deep or extensive burn may need to be debrided, a process that cleanses the area and removes dead skin. This is a procedure that must be done by a medical professional.

■ Depending on the depth and extent of the burn, your doctor may recommend that your child be given a tetanus shot and/or an antibiotic, such as penicillin, to guard against infection.

■ The physician may dress the area with a bandage that contains a film of a topical antibiotic, such as silver sulfadiazine (Silvadene).

■ Your doctor may prescribe an antibiotic ointment for dressing your child's burn at home. Antibiotic ointments such as Silvadene, povidone-iodine (Betadine), gentamicin sulfate, and bacitracin are used to treat an existing infection or to prevent one from developing. Your doctor will instruct you to apply a thin layer of ointment over the burned area, and to cover it with sterile gauze. There are also a number of new "high-tech" dressings available that can be left on for days at a time. These are especially suitable for milder burns. Ask your doctor about this.

■ Any burn that affects the mouth should be treated promptly by a doctor or pediatric dentist to ensure that it heals properly, without inflicting permanent damage. In some cases, a special appliance may be necessary to prevent the wound from contracting as it heals, leaving a child with a condition known as *microsomia* (literally, small mouth).

GENERAL RECOMMENDATIONS

■ If your child suffers a serious burn, take appropriate emergency measures. Rely on medical personnel to treat the injury properly.

■ If your child suffers a minor burn, promptly cool the area under cool running water to minimize damage. Once the area has cooled, apply aloe vera gel and continue applying three times a day until the wound has healed.

■ Do not use ice water directly on a burn. Doing so can deepen and worsen the burn. Instead use cool compresses or running water.

■ Never apply butter, petroleum jelly, ointment, or cream to a burn. A greasy substance will trap the heat and cause a burn to deepen.

■ Do not bandage or cover the affected area tightly. A tight covering traps the heat and can cause a burn to deepen.

■ Do not break any blisters. They form a natural bandage that aids healing.

■ After proper emergency treatment has been administered, give your child the herb gotu kola—one dose, three times a day, for one to two weeks following a burn. This herb helps heal skin tissue.

Caution: Do not give gotu kola to a child under four years of age.

■ To help lessen the stinging and pain of a burn, give your child the homeopathic *Urtica urens* 12x or 6c, every 15 minutes, up to four doses. You can also apply topical *Urtica urens* ointment or gel to the burn.

■ Giving your child nutritional supplements of vitamin C, bioflavonoids, vitamin E, and zinc will help the skin heal.

Choking

According to the American Academy of Pediatrics, children under four years of age are at the greatest risk of choking, not only on small, removable parts of toys—a danger most parents guard against—but on food as well. In 1991, the National Safety Council reported that 270 American children four years old and under died as a result of choking on food. Consumer advocates are now lobbying to have labels warning of possible choking hazards placed on certain food products that are popular with children.

A study published in a 1995 issue of the *Journal of the American Medical Association* found that balloons are the most common cause of death from choking in children less than three years old. In fact, the accompanying article further stated that with the exception of bicycles and other riding toys, balloons cause more deaths in children than any other toy.

It's frightening to realize that your child is choking. First, make a quick assessment of the situation. If your child is talking or coughing forcefully, you do not need to intervene. This indicates that air is getting through the windpipe. As long as your child can breathe, she may be able to expel the material on her own. Watch and wait. A child's coughing and sputtering is often enough to expel the object.

However, if your child becomes unable to speak, makes frantic, high-pitched sounds, gasps for air, turns blue, or clutches at her throat, act fast. Your child needs emergency help.

The Heimlich maneuver, developed by Dr. H. J. Heimlich, is the emergency treatment procedure we endorse for a choking child. Guidelines for both a child over one year old and an infant under one year old are provided, beginning on the next page.

Be aware that the American Heart Association and the American Red Cross teach a different procedure for treating a choking infant under one year old. They advise the following: Sit down and hold the baby securely, resting face down on your forearm. Using the heel of your hand, give your baby 5 quick, firm blows between his shoulder blades. Turn the baby over to face you, then with your fingers, give 5 quick, firm compressions to his breastbone just below the nipple line. Look for foreign material in the baby's mouth. If you see anything, remove it, but do not blindly sweep your finger through his mouth. Repeat these steps until the foreign material is expelled.

While this method is widely taught, there has been concern that a back slap can cause the foreign object to lodge even deeper in the throat. And chest and abdominal thrusts have been known to cause broken ribs and damaged organs.

After careful research, it is the opinion of the authors of this book, that the Heimlich maneuver is the safest, most effective procedure for children of all ages, including infants.

The information in this entry cannot substitute for a certified first aid class in which you can learn and practice the Heimlich maneuver. Rather, it is intended to serve as a refresher in case of an emergency.

EMERGENCY TREATMENT FOR CHOKING

✚ Have someone call for emergency help and go to your child's aid quickly. Your child's age will determine the measures you must take to relieve choking. Perform the age-appropriate procedure outlined below. **Do not stop** until the foreign material is expelled, **or** your child begins coughing, breathing, and making normal sounds on her own, **or** another person can take over for you, **or** medical help arrives.

For a Choking Infant Under One Year Old

The Heimlich maneuver should be performed on an infant under one year old as follows:

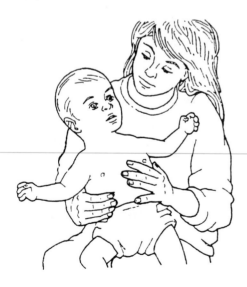

1. Sit on a chair and place your baby on your lap facing away from you.

For a Choking Child Over One Year Old

The Heimlich maneuver should be performed on a child over one year old as follows:

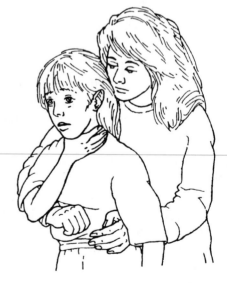

1. Stand or kneel behind your child, wrapping your arms around her waist.

94

For a Choking Infant Under One Year Old

For a Choking Child Over One Year Old

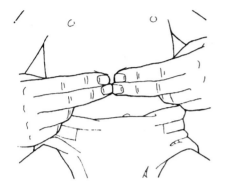

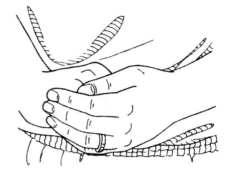

2. Put the tips of both of your index and middle fingers together to form one compression pad. Position this "pad" against your baby's abdomen, above the navel and just below the rib cage.

2. Make a fist with one hand and clasp your other hand over your fist. Position the thumb side of your fist against your child's abdomen, just above the navel and below the rib cage.

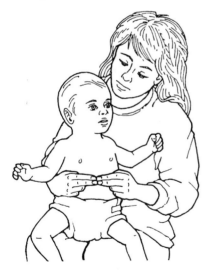

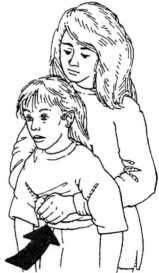

3. Use a gentle, quick, *upward* push of your fingers into your baby's abdomen to force air up through the windpipe.

3. Use a quick, forceful, *upward* push of your fist into your child's abdomen to force air up through the windpipe.

4. Continue doing these thrusts until your baby expels the foreign material.

4. Continue doing these thrusts until your child expels the foreign material.

For a Choking Infant Under One Year Old

If your baby loses consciousness, discontinue the thrusts and open her airway as follows:

5. Look for foreign material in your baby's mouth. If you see anything, remove it, but **do not** blindly sweep your finger through her mouth.

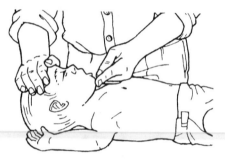

6. Tip your baby's head back by pushing on her forehead. With your other hand, gently lift the bony part of the jaw. This opens the airway.

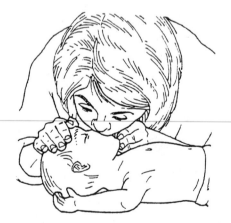

7. Cover your baby's nose and mouth with your mouth and give 2 gentle puffs of air, just enough to make your her chest rise and fall as in normal breathing.

For a Choking Child Over One Year Old

If your child loses consciousness, discontinue the thrusts and open her airway as follows:

5. Look for foreign material in your child's mouth. If you see anything, remove it, but **do not** blindly sweep your finger through her mouth.

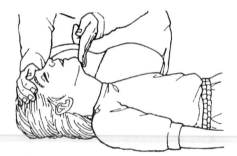

6. Tip your child's head back by pushing on her forehead. With your other hand, gently lift the bony part of the jaw. This opens the airway.

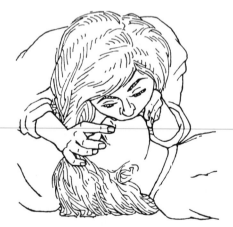

7. Pinch your child's nostrils closed. Cover her mouth with yours and give 2 slow breaths of air, just enough to make her chest rise and fall as in normal breathing.

For a Choking Infant Under One Year Old

If her chest is not rising and falling when you give the breaths, the airway is still blocked. You will have to try again to dislodge the foreign material.

8. Repeat steps 1 through 4 until the material is expelled, *or* your baby begins coughing, breathing, and making normal sounds on her own, *or* another person can take over for you, *or* emergency help arrives.

For a Choking Child Over One Year Old

If her chest is not rising and falling when you give the breaths, the airway is still blocked. You will have to try again to dislodge the foreign material.

8. Repeat steps 1 through 4 until the material is expelled, *or* your child begins coughing, breathing, and making normal sounds on her own, *or* another person can take over for you, *or* emergency help arrives.

✚ Even if your child seems to be fine once the material has been expelled, she should be seen by a doctor to be checked for possible damage to her windpipe or abdomen.

GENERAL RECOMMENDATIONS

■ After emergency treatment has been administered and the crisis is over, give your child Bach Flower Rescue Remedy—three drops, three times a day, for one week. Rescue Remedy will help to ease any fear, panic, anxiety, or tension.

■ Give your child a cup of slippery elm tea or a combination of ⅔ slippery elm and ⅓ licorice root. This will help soothe the throat.
Caution: Do not give licorice to a child with high blood pressure.

PREVENTION

■ Infants and very young children explore the world around them by putting anything and everything into their mouths. Keep a close watch. Teach your child never to put any object into her mouth except for the food you provide.

■ Young children should always be supervised when eating.

■ When preparing a meal or snack for a young child, cut all foods, including fruits, into very small pieces, and offer one bite at a time. Even a cookie, graham cracker, or banana can pose a risk. A young child who doesn't chew well may try to swallow a sticky, too-large "gummed" bite of food. According to the American Academy of Pediatrics, the following child-pleasing foods are particularly dangerous to children under four:

- thick "sticky" candies
- hard candies
- raw carrots
- celery
- grapes and raisins
- hot dogs
- chunks of meat
- lumps of peanut butter
- popcorn
- nuts

■ Eat slowly and chew thoroughly, and teach your child to do the same. A child in a rush to finish a meal can choke on a poorly chewed or extra-large bite of food.

■ Select toys that are well made and appropriate for your child's age. Examine your child's toys and playthings regularly to make sure that all small parts are secure.

■ For suggestions on how to childproof your home and minimize hazards your child may encounter outside, *see* HOME SAFETY in Part One.

Concussion (Head Injury)

Any injury to your child's head, whether from falling off a swing, getting banged on the monkey bars, being hit by a flying object, or being jarred or shaken violently, may result in a concussion. It is rare for a child to reach adulthood without ever experiencing a hard knock on the head from one cause or another. The severity of your child's symptoms will depend on the extent of injury to the brain.

After a simple concussion, your child may seem disoriented or lose consciousness briefly. She may have no memory of events just prior to and immediately following the injury. Headaches, dizziness, and drowsiness are all common immediately after awakening. Such symptoms usually disappear within a few weeks, but can last as long as several months.

If your child suffers a head injury, watch her closely afterward. If any of the following symptoms occurs, even as much as four weeks after a seemingly mild bang on the head, seek medical attention immediately, as these can be signs of bleeding in the brain:

- Loss of consciousness.
- Unusually widened pupils.
- Severe headache.
- Drowsiness.
- Personality changes.
- Confusion; loss of memory; speech difficulties.
- Loss of coordination; paralysis.

EMERGENCY TREATMENT FOR CONCUSSION

✚ After any injury to the head, it is wise to call your physician or take your child to the emergency room of the nearest hospital. It is important to seek the advice of a qualified medical professional. The severity of head injuries is difficult for the layperson to evaluate, and head injuries are one of the most common causes of death in children.

CONVENTIONAL TREATMENT

■ Seek medical help immediately. The doctor will examine your child and possibly order an x-ray of her skull to check for a fracture, or a magnetic resonance imaging (MRI) scan to look for bleeding or swelling in the brain. Be prepared to answer questions about your child's reaction right after the accident, including any unusual behavior. The doctor will evaluate your child's condition and provide appropriate treatment.

■ Your doctor will probably recommend that you keep close watch on your child for a minimum of twenty-four hours after returning home.

GENERAL RECOMMENDATIONS

■ After emergency treatment has been administered and the crisis is over, give your child Bach Flower Rescue Remedy—three drops, three times a day, for one week. Rescue Remedy will help to ease any fear, panic, anxiety, or tension.

■ In addition to Rescue Remedy, give your child one dose of homeopathic *Aconite* 30c immediately after the crisis (and after evaluation by a doctor or professional health care provider) to help easy any fright.

Consciousness, Loss of

See FAINTING; UNCONSCIOUSNESS.

Convulsion

See SEIZURE.

Cuts and Scrapes

Cuts, scrapes, and skinned knees and elbows are an inevitable part of childhood. Because any break in the skin can become infected, even minor injuries should be treated fairly aggressively. A child's skin is thin and delicate. Also, whereas an adult body has had decades to develop infection-fighting antibodies, your child has not yet developed a full storehouse of the antibodies that fight skin bacteria.

Cuts and scrapes on the head, face, hands, mouth, and feet can bleed profusely, because there are many blood vessels close to the surface of the skin in these areas. To avoid scarring, you'll want to treat a cut on your child's face especially carefully. Cuts on the face, fingers, and hands are particularly vulnerable to infection because they are not covered with clothing. Cuts involving the lips should be inspected by a doctor. Stitches may be required to ensure that your child's mouth heals normally.

You can treat minor cuts and scrapes at home with basic first aid. However, occasions may arise when medical care is essential. If you have any doubt about your ability to care for a child's injury properly, consult your doctor.

EMERGENCY TREATMENT
FOR CUTS AND SCRAPES

✚ If your child's wound is caused by a dirty or rusty object, or if there is foreign material embedded in the wound, take your child to the doctor promptly. A serious infection could result. Also, your child may require a tetanus shot.

✚ If bleeding does not stop within ten to fifteen minutes, if the edges of the skin are separated and the wound is open, or if the wound is deep or extensive, see your doctor. Your child may require stitches, which can help prevent infection, hasten healing, and make any scar that results small and barely noticeable.

CONVENTIONAL TREATMENT

■ The first step in treating any wound is to cleanse and disinfect the site. For a minor cut or scrape, you can do this at home. If the injury is more serious, your child's physician can do it. If a wound is severe or dirty, your doctor may administer a tetanus shot, especially if it has been more than five years since your child last had one.

■ Depending on the extent of the wound, your child's doctor may close a cut with stitches or a butterfly adhesive bandage. If you are treating a minor cut at home, cover it with an adhesive bandage. A wound that is covered is less likely to become infected.

■ To prevent infection, over-the-counter antibiotic ointments such as Neosporin, Betadine, or bacitracin are often recommended.

GENERAL RECOMMENDATIONS

■ To stop bleeding, apply firm pressure to the wound with a piece of sterile gauze or a clean cloth. Putting ice on the cut will also help stop bleeding, because cold constricts blood vessels and slows blood flow. If your child's mouth or tongue is cut, try using a fruit-juice popsicle.

■ Cleansing is the cornerstone of treatment for any break in the skin. Wash your child's wound with generous amounts of water. Thoroughly clean out any particles of dirt or foreign matter that may have gotten into the cut by holding the wound under running water. Be sure the wound is cleaned well immediately after the injury, and keep the area scrupulously clean while it is still open and healing.

■ If your child's cut is deeper than a scratch, cover it with gauze or an adhesive bandage. A superficial scratch can be left open to the air.

■ Cover the wound with the ointment of your choice to speed healing. Calendula ointment or gel is an antiseptic and anti-inflammatory. Comfrey salve helps speed wound healing. Topical aloe vera is good for its soothing and healing properties.

■ Raw, unprocessed honey is a natural antiseptic that can be applied directly to a wound. It is especially helpful when no other treatments are readily available.

Diarrhea

Diarrhea, or frequent and watery stools, is the body's way of ridding itself of toxins and foreign substances. Most cases of simple diarrhea should not be suppressed too quickly. It may be healthier to allow your child's body to flush itself clean, while supporting her with adequate fluids.

There are many microorganisms that can cause diarrhea, including viruses, bacteria, fungi, and protozoa. Your child can pick up viruses, bacteria, or protozoa from other children, or from contaminated food and water. Food poisoning causes diarrhea very quickly. A milk allergy or food sensitivity, which may surface with the introduction of new foods, can also cause diarrhea.

Less common causes of diarrhea include reactions to medication, inflammatory bowel disease, hepatitis, cystic fibrosis, and pancreatitis. An anatomical deformity such as a fistula, or a congenital defect such as Hirschsprung's disease or short bowel syndrome, can also cause diarrhea. If your child's diarrhea arises from any of these conditions, she requires medical attention.

Most cases of simple diarrhea are caused by viruses. Viruses invade a child's intestinal tract, causing irritation and inflammation of the intestinal walls. Viruses also induce the cells that line the intestines to secrete fluids. The increase in fluid volume in turn increases peristalsis, the wavelike contractions of the intestines. The result is cramping and the loose, watery, frequent stools characteristic of diarrhea.

Vomiting and stomachache often accompany diarrhea, and abdominal cramps usually come and go, often occurring right before a bowel movement. Depending on the cause of the diarrhea, a fever may or may not be present. When a child is suffering from diarrhea, dehydration is always a serious concern, especially if her temperature is elevated. In the first two or three months of life, an infant can become dehydrated very quickly, so if your newborn develops diarrhea, call your physician.

Watching for signs of dehydration is the most important tool you can use when assessing the child's level of illness or health. Signs of dehydration include a dry mouth, decreased urination, increased thirst, cool, dry skin, and a mildly elevated temperature. More signs of advanced dehydration include listlessness, sunken eyes, sunken fontanels in infants, and no tears.

Observe your child between episodes of diarrhea to get a sense of how sick she is. If your child is alert and not experiencing cramping between episodes, it's safe to assume her body probably has the situation under control. But if your child seems weak and the cramping is not relieved between episodes, call your health care provider.

WHEN TO CALL THE DOCTOR
ABOUT DIARRHEA

• In newborns, diarrhea is signaled by an increase in stools, stools that are unusually loose or watery, stools that are yellowish or greenish in color, or stools with a foul odor. Always consult a doctor about a newborn's diarrhea.

• If your child experiences severe or persistent abdominal pain with diarrhea, or has blood in the stool, call your doctor right away.

• If your child has a case of diarrhea that lasts for longer than forty-eight hours, or intermittent diarrhea that comes and goes over a period of one week or longer, seek the advice of your health care practitioner.

• Vomiting that accompanies gastrointestinal upsets should not last for more than twenty-four hours. Call your doctor if your child has been experiencing diarrhea with vomiting for longer than that.

CONVENTIONAL TREATMENT

■ To prevent dehydration, oral electrolyte formulas, such as Pedialyte, Lytren, Ricelyte, and Resol, are commonly recommended for children with diarrhea.

■ Loperamide (sold as Imodium AD tablets and liquid) is the most commonly used antidiarrheal, now that it is available over the counter. It acts by slowing the movement of the intestinal muscle.

Caution: You should never give your child loperamide if she has a fever over 101°F or bloody stools. This drug is not recommended for children under twelve.

■ Kaolin-pectin, an over-the-counter drug better known as Kaopectate, binds substances in the intestines with excess water, thereby solidifying and drying diarrheal stools. This makes it appear as if your child is having less diarrhea and more formed stools, but she is actually losing the same amount of water as she would be if untreated. It just looks different. Kaolin medications can give a false sense of reassurance.

■ Bismuth subsalicylate (Pepto-Bismol) is an over-the-counter drug that works by attaching to the toxin or bacteria that is causing the problem in the intestines. This deactivates the foreign substance and it loses its ability to hurt the body. This medication can turn the stools black. It is not recommended for children under two years of age and should not be taken with products that contain aspirin.

■ Antibiotics can help, but only if your child's diarrhea is due to a parasitic or bacterial infection. They should be prescribed only after a stool analysis or culture confirms this.

■ Antidiarrheal medications that contain opiates, such as paregoric and Lomotil, are not recommended for children. Like loperamide, these drugs work by slowing down intestinal action and halting bowel movements. But these are powerful drugs that contain narcotics, and are not necessarily safe.

GENERAL RECOMMENDATIONS

■ Be sure your child is taking adequate fluids. When a small body is losing fluids as rapidly as it does with diarrhea, dehydration is a very serious concern. If you are not comfortable with the progress your child is making, do not hesitate to consult your doctor.

Rehydration Formula

The following rehydration formula is helpful for both children and adults.

1 teaspoon salt
1 cup powdered rice cereal
1 quart water

1. In a small bowl, combine the ingredients well.
2. Give your child 1 teaspoon of the formula every 15 minutes.
3. Keep the formula covered and refrigerated.
4. Make a new batch every 12 hours.

■ If your child is vomiting in addition to having diarrhea, even a small sip of water may cause another upset. If vomiting occurs after your child takes water, wait one hour and then offer small chips of ice. If the vomiting reflex is not triggered by the ice, after an hour of calm has passed, offer more chips of ice or small sips of water. Or, as an alternative, try giving your child a teaspoon of Emetrol syrup or raw honey to settle her stomach.

Caution: Never give honey to a child less than one year old. Honey has been associated with infant botulism, which can be life threatening.

■ *Do not* offer your child food until she signals a readiness to eat. If your child is hungry, give her simple, easily digested foods. Avoid dairy products, which may be difficult to digest.

■ If done properly, rehydrating with sips of water can be just as effective as intravenous hydration done in the hospital. The important thing is to give frequent sips of fluid; for example, give 1 teaspoon of liquid every 15 minutes. Be careful not to give too much at one time so as not to induce vomiting. A child older than one year can be given raw honey, barley malt, or rice bran syrup mixed with water. These mixtures are a source of calories and will help settle the stomach. Miso soup and diluted fruit juices are also good liquids to help keep a child hydrated. A great rehydration formula for all ages contains 1 teaspoon of salt, 1 cup of powdered rice cereal, and 1 quart of water. Give 1 teaspoon of this formula every 15 minutes. Make a fresh batch every 12 hours.

■ In addition to the conventional treatments for diarrhea, the homeopathic *Arsenicum album* is helpful in easing diarrhea brought on by food poisoning, anxiety, or stress. Give your child *Arsenicum album* 30c—one dose every two hours, for six hours.

■ The Chinese formula Curing Pills (in liquid form), will help ease most stomach or intestinal upsets including diarrhea. Goldenseal is also helpful due to its astringent, antiviral, and antibacterial properties.

■ Charcoal tablets will help absorb toxins in the large intestine.
Caution: Do not give charcoal to a child under 8 years old.

PREVENTION

■ To prevent bacteria and foreign substances from finding their way into your child's system, teach your child to wash her hands properly after going to the bathroom and before eating.

■ Try to eliminate any food allergies or sensitivities as a cause of diarrhea. Common allergens include citrus fruits, wheat, sugar, and dairy products.

■ If your child suffers repeated bouts of diarrhea, she may have a lactose intolerance. The absorption of lactose, or milk sugar, depends on the presence of the enzyme lactase. Most infants have adequate amounts of this enzyme, but older children and adults often don't produce enough of it to process lactose. As a result, they suffer from diarrhea, bloating, vague abdominal pain, gas, and indigestion when they consume dairy products. About 33 million people in the United States are lactose intolerant. The most effective treatment for this condition is to limit the intake of milk and dairy products, as well as processed food products that contain lactose as an ingredient.

Drowning, Near

A child of any age, even a good swimmer, can suffer a water accident that causes a near-drowning. It can happen even in very shallow water. In fact, a 1985 article in *Emergency Medical Review* noted that 90 percent of all drownings occur within ten yards of land. The biggest danger of drowning comes from a lack of oxygen. Cardiac arrest as a result of immersion in cold water can also be a cause of death in drowning. Complications of a near-drowning can include damage to internal organs, especially the brain, due to lack of oxygen, and damage to the lungs from inhaling water, salt, sand, or bacteria.

EMERGENCY TREATMENT FOR NEAR-DROWNING

✚ If your child is thrashing around in a panic or is unconscious, go into the water after her (if you are not a good swimmer, take a life preserver with you). Check for breathing as soon as you reach your child, while you are still in the water.

✚ If your child is not breathing, you must breathe for her immediately. Don't waste time getting your child out of the water first, and don't worry about getting the water out of her lungs. Begin rescue breathing immediately, in the manner appropriate for your child's age, as you carry her out of the water (turn to CARDIOPULMONARY RESUSCITATION on page 33). Maintain artificial respiration continuously until emergency personnel arrive, until you can get your child to the emergency room of the nearest hospital, or until your child begins breathing on her own. Don't panic, and don't become discouraged and give up prematurely. Victims of near-drowning with barely perceptible pulses have been successfully revived when artificial respiration was steadily maintained for an extended period of time.

✚ Once your child is breathing and out of the water, drain as much water as possible from her lungs. Hold your child around the waist, allowing her trunk and head to hang down (*see* figure). Sometimes just holding a child in this position is sufficient to expel inhaled water. If your child begins coughing and sputtering, and struggles to reach an upright position, you may safely

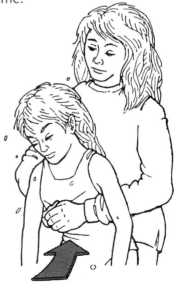

assume that the initial crisis has passed. She will still need medical attention to detect and treat any possible complications.

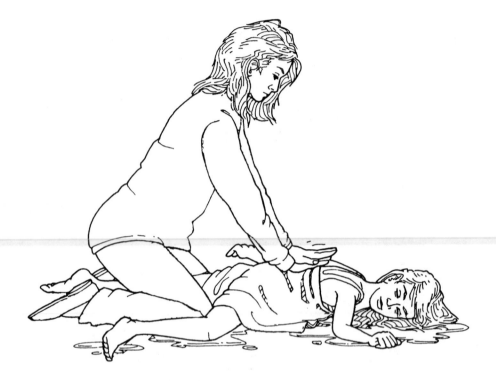

✚ If your child is breathing on her own, but the procedure on page 107 fails to expel water from the lungs, try the following. Place her on her stomach, with the leg and arm on one side of her body straight out, the hand palm side up. On the other side of the body, position the leg with the knee bent and drawn up toward the body at a right angle, and the arm with elbow bent and drawn toward the chest, the hand palm side flat to the ground. Turn her head toward the side with the bent limbs, with her jaw jutting slightly forward to open the airway.

Then, with the heels of your hands, press down on the upper quadrant of the back to compress the lungs and force any inhaled water up through the windpipe, or trachea. If there is water in your child's lungs, it should gush out, initiating coughing and sputtering. If paramedics are not already on their way to you, seek medical attention immediately.

✚ After a near-drowning, even if your child seems to be fine, she should be examined by a doctor.

GENERAL RECOMMENDATIONS

■ After emergency treatment has been administered and the crisis is over, give your child Bach Flower Rescue Remedy—three drops, three times a day, for one week. Rescue Remedy will help to ease any fear, panic, anxiety, or tension.

■ In addition to Rescue Remedy, give your child one dose of the homeopathic *Aconite* 30c to help ease any fright. This will also help alleviate any shivering or chills.

PREVENTION

■ Make sure your child learns to swim and learns water safety.

■ Do not permit your child to jump into deep water unless there is an easy way for her to get out again, such as a ladder on the side of a pool, or a nearby bank with a shallow slope. A child who jumps into deep water from the side of a boat, the edge of a cliff, or a steep bank may be difficult to rescue in case of an accident.

■ Always outfit your child with a suitable life jacket when she is engaged in any activity in or on the water, including boating, sailing, and windsurfing, even if she is a good swimmer.

■ Allow your child to swim in pools or at public beaches only if a lifeguard is on duty.

■ Always make sure your child is supervised by a responsible adult when she is around water, including bathtime. *Never* leave a child alone in the tub or near water.

■ Do not permit your child to walk or slide on an iced-over pond, river, creek, or lake unless the ice has been thoroughly tested by a responsible adult.

■ When enjoying water sports with your child, don't drink alcoholic beverages. Alcohol impairs your reflexes and could keep you from acting quickly and surely enough to help your child if a crisis arises.

Drug Overdose

See POISONING.

Electric Shock

A severe electric shock may knock your child unconscious, and he may stop breathing. There may be deep burns at the point where the current entered the body. There may also be internal damage.

EMERGENCY TREATMENT
FOR ELECTRIC SHOCK

✚ You will probably instinctively reach to snatch your child out of harm's way. **Don't.** You may receive a severe shock yourself and become unable to help your child. To break the electrical contact safely, first switch off the current. If this is not possible, as in the case of a live wire, use a nonconductive item, such as a wooden broom handle, to lift or push away the source of the current.

✚ *If your child is not breathing and has no pulse, turn to* CARDIOPUL-MONARY RESUSCITATION (CPR) *on page 33. Start artificial respiration at once.*

✚ Always take your child to the doctor or the emergency room for evaluation after a severe electric shock, even if he seems to have suffered only a minor burn. There may be internal damage.

CONVENTIONAL TREATMENT

■ If your child has suffered a burn as a result of an electric shock, *see* the entry on BURNS for appropriate treatment suggestions.

GENERAL RECOMMENDATIONS

■ After emergency treatment has been given and the crisis is over, give your child Bach Flower Rescue Remedy—three drops, three times a day, for one week. Rescue Remedy will help ease any fear, panic, anxiety, or tension.

■ In addition to Rescue Remedy, give your child one dose of homeopathic *Aconite* 30c, every hour, for three hours. *Aconite* is helpful in easing physical symptoms that are intense, come on suddenly, and are associated with fright. Follow with *Arnica* 30c one dose, three times a day, for one day.

Epileptic Seizure

See SEIZURE.

Eye Injuries

Eye injuries can be the result of a blow or blunt trauma, a laceration, a chemical burn, or an embedded object. Even a small foreign particle, such as an eyelash or cinder, if not properly removed, can damage the eye. Any type of injury to the eye can be serious and should be treated as such. Even if there appears to be no obvious damage to the area, it is wise to have any eye injury evaluated by an ophthalmologist.

Common signs and symptoms of an injured eye include a visible bruise or cut, pain in or around the eye, sensitivity to light, the inability to keep the eye open, constant tearing, blurred or impaired vision, rapid blinking, and headache.

EMERGENCY TREATMENT
FOR EYE INJURIES

Follow the appropriate steps outlined below for the specific eye injury your child has suffered.

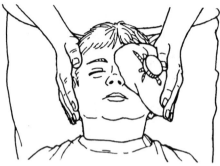

✚ For a Black Eye:

1. Place a cold compress or ice pack over—but not directly on—the bruised eye. Leave the compress on for 10 to 15 minute intervals. This will help reduce pain and swelling. ***Avoid excessive pressure on the eyelid.***

2. It may be necessary to have a doctor evaluate the injury to be sure there is no damage to the eye or fracture to the facial bones or skull.

3. If your child wakes up with a black eye and there is no apparent explanation, have him evaluated by a doctor. This could be a symptom of an underlying illness.

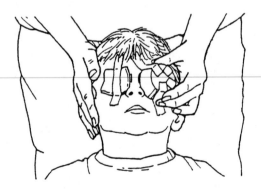

✚ For an Embedded Object:

1. Immediately call 911 or take the child to the nearest hospital emergency room.

2. ***Do not touch or press the embedded object or try to remove it.***

3. Have the child lie as still as possible on his back.

4. To keep a large object, such as a stick or pencil, from moving and causing further damage, support the object by placing a paper cup over the eye and taping it in place. You may have to poke a hole in the bottom of the cup to let the object through. ***Do not touch the eye.*** To prevent further movement, cover the child's other eye with a sterile pad or clean cloth and tape it in place.

5. For a small embedded object, cover both eyes with sterile pads or clean cloths and loosely tape them in place.

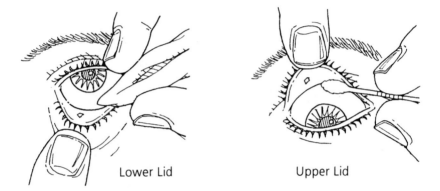

Lower Lid   Upper Lid

✚ For a Foreign Object that is not Embedded:

1. To remove a small object, such as a cinder or eyelash, have your child look up while you gently pull down his lower eyelid. If you see the object, gently pull the child's upper eyelid down over his lower eyelid. This will produce tears, which may flush the object from the eye.

2. If the tears do not flush out the object, try to rinse it out with lukewarm water. (You might also have the child try opening his eyes in a bowl of fresh water.) If you see the object, you can try lifting it off with the corner of a clean damp cloth or cotton swab.

3. If you do not see the object inside the lower eyelid, have you child look down while you gently lift his upper eyelid. If you see the object, either flush it out with lukewarm water or lift it off with the corner of a clean, damp cloth or cotton swab.

4. If you cannot remove the object, cover both of the child's eyes with sterile pads or clean cloths and loosely tape them in place.

5. Take the child to the nearest emergency facility.

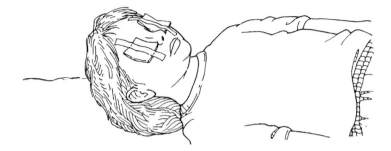

✚ For a Scratched or Cut Eye:

1. Rinse the scratched eye with clean, cool water for several minutes. You can use the water from a faucet, a pitcher, or a glass.

2. Cover both eyes with sterile pads or clean cloths and loosely tape them into place. ***Do not apply any pressure.***

3. Take the child to the nearest emergency facility.

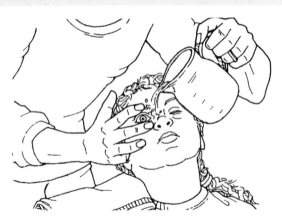

✚ For Chemical in the Eye:

1. Hold your child's eyelids apart and flush the affected eye with clean, lukewarm water for 20 to 30 minutes. You can use the water from a faucet, a pitcher, or a glass. While flushing, be sure the affected eye is lower than the other one. (This will prevent any chemical from splashing into the uninjured eye.)

2. Cover both eyes with sterile pads or clean cloths and loosely tape them into place. ***Do not apply any pressure.***

3. Take the child to the nearest emergency facility.

CONVENTIONAL TREATMENT

■ For a bruised or black eye, an ophthalmologist will perform a thorough examination to assess any damage to the internal structures of the eye and the facial bones. Surgery may be required.

■ Before removing a foreign object from the eye, the doctor may apply a topical anesthetic to minimize the pain.

■ The doctor may place fluorescein into an injured eye. This dye enables the doctor to clearly see any scratches or small injuries on the eye's surface.

■ Depending on the severity and type of eye injury, the doctor may prescribe an antibiotic cream or pill to help prevent infection.

GENERAL RECOMMENDATIONS

■ For a bruised or black eye, use ice packs or cold compresses to help reduce swelling and alleviate pain.

■ Once emergency treatments have been administered and the crisis is over, give your child homeopathic *Arnica* and *Ledum* to help heal the bruising and tissue trauma. Give one dose of *Arnica* 30c followed an hour later by one dose of *Ledum* 30c. Continue giving *Ledum* 30c, three times a day, for two days.

■ Following a mild eye injury, a diluted eyewash containing the herb eyebright is soothing and cleansing. Do not use this if the eye has been punctured or has a laceration.

Fainting

See also UNCONSCIOUSNESS.

Fainting—medically termed *syncope* (sin'-ka-pee)— is a sudden and temporary loss of consciousness that occurs as a result of a lack of blood flow to the brain. There are a number of things that can cause this to occur, including a sudden drop in blood pressure, anemia, epilepsy, extreme heat, breath-holding and hyperventilation, hunger, and hypoglycemia. Standing for a long time in a hot, stuffy room, exhaustion, emotional upset, fear, or fever may also cause a child to faint.

In the moments before a fainting episode, a child may experience dizziness, weakness, and a feeling of numbness in the hands or feet; he may suddenly turn pale and his skin may feel cold. Upon awakening, he may feel tired and develop a headache.

If a child loses consciousness apparently due to one of the factors listed above and makes a complete recovery within fifteen minutes, it is likely that he has experienced a fainting episode. A child who has fainted will usually awaken fairly readily, especially if you use smelling salts, and will be aware and oriented upon awakening.

If you find a child unconscious and have not actually seen him faint, or if he regained consciousness with difficulty and is disoriented, it is possible that he has a more serious problem. Turn to UNCONSCIOUSNESS on page 173.

EMERGENCY TREATMENT FOR FAINTING

✚ If you see your child lose consciousness, take the following measures immediately:

1. Check for pulse and breathing. **If pulse and/or breathing are absent, or if either stops at any time during the episode, turn to CARDIOPULMONARY RESUSCITATION on page 33.** Begin taking the appropriate measures at once.

2. If the child is breathing and his heart rate seems to be fine, check for signs of injury. If the child is unknown to you, look to see if he is wearing a Medic Alert bracelet that offers an explanation for the episode, such as a history of diabetes or epilepsy.

3. If there are no signs of injury, try the following, in order, to provoke a response:

   • Call the child's name.

   • Pat his face gently.

   • Wave smelling salts under his nose. If smelling salts are not readily available, try using an open bottle of perfume.

   • **Do not** splash cold water on your child's face. **Do not** shake your child.

4. If the child is still limp and unresponsive, lay him flat with his feet elevated, or head lowered, to a 45-degree angle if possible. This will increase the

flow of blood to the brain. Loosen his clothing. If the child begins to vomit, place him in the recovery position by rolling him on his side (*see* below). This will ensure that the child's airway will not be obstructed. (If you suspect a head or neck injury, *see* IMMOBILIZING AN INJURED HEAD, NECK, AND BACK, beginning on page 44.) Cover him with a blanket or sweater so that he stays warm. Stay with your child and continue to monitor his pulse and breathing.

5. If he does not regain consciousness within two or three minutes, or if his pulse or breathing becomes weaker, call for emergency help.

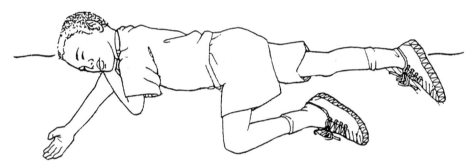

The Recovery Position

✚ Once the child regains consciousness, help him into a sitting position. Have him lean forward, with his head between his knees, to increase blood circulation to the brain.

✚ Have your child lie still for an additional ten to fifteen minutes after he has recovered from the episode, to be sure he is stable enough to walk.

✚ Call your doctor and explain the situation. A child who has experienced a fainting episode should be examined by a physician.

GENERAL RECOMMENDATIONS

■ If your child feels faint, place a cool washcloth on the back of his neck.

■ To help prevent a fainting episode, have your child sit up and place his head between his knees.

■ Pressing hard on the acupressure point called the Governing Vessel 21, located directly under the nose (*see* below), can sometimes prevent a fainting episode.

■ Once your child has regained consciousness after a fainting episode and the crisis is over, give him one dose of Bach Flower Rescue Remedy to help ease any fear, panic, anxiety, or tension.

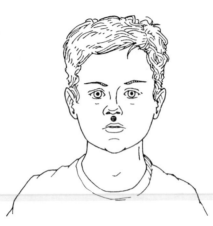

Governing Vessel 21

Fever

When taken by mouth, a child's body temperature is usually between 96.8°F and 99.4°F (36°C to 37.2°C). A child's temperature normally varies by as much as 2°F, depending on his level of activity, emotional stress, the amount of clothing worn, the time of day, and the temperature of the environment, among other factors.

A fever can be caused by a wide variety of things, including dehydration, overexertion, mosquito bites, bee stings, an allergic or toxic reaction, or a viral or bacterial infection. Fever of unknown origin (FUO) is a condition defined as an elevated temperature lasting for a week or more without an identifiable cause. Fever in and of itself is not necessarily harmful.

In most cases, a fever is the body's reaction to an acute viral or bacterial infection. It is not necessarily a dangerous condition. Rather, it is a sign that the body is defending itself against the infectious invader. Since viruses and bacteria do not survive as well in a body with an elevated temperature, fever is actually an ally in fighting infection. It is one of the ways in which the body defends and heals itself. An elevated temperature also increases the production of infection-fighting white blood cells and even increases their speed of response and enhances their killing capacity.

In an adult, the level of fever generally reflects the severity of the illness causing it. In a child, however, this is not necessarily the case. A child with a mild cold may have a 105°F fever, while a child with a serious illness—bacterial pneumonia, for example—may have only a 100°F fever.

In a newborn, the body's temperature control is not yet well developed. As a result, signs other than a fever—poor appetite, lethargy, and irritability—may be earlier indicators of an infection and therefore more helpful than temperature in assessing your newborn's condition. However, when a newborn has an elevated or low temperature, he should be examined by a doctor.

When assessing your child's condition, the most important thing to do is to observe how your child is acting. How sick does your child seem to you? A child with a fever may be pale or flushed, feel hot to the touch, and have dry or sweaty skin. He may feel restless, achy, unable to sleep, and unwilling to eat. Be aware of other symptoms that accompany your child's fever. If a feverish child has red spots on his skin, a runny nose, and eyes that are red and perhaps more sensitive to light than usual, he may be getting measles. If a child has a fever and red, itchy spots on his body, he may be coming down with chickenpox. A baby with a fever in combination with a reddish-pink rash and swollen glands in his neck may have roseola.

If a child over one year old has a slight fever, no intervention may be necessary. Unless your child's temperature is higher than 102°F, fever-reducing medication is generally not needed. However, a child with an elevated temperature may be very uncomfortable. A feverish child typically doesn't rest or desire food. His whole body aches. A fever raises the child's overall metabolic rate. When his metabolism is racing, your child can easily lose weight and body fluids. Gently bringing a fever down can help your child feel better and help to prevent complications, such as dehydration.

Bringing down a fever can also help indicate the severity of your child's illness and aid in diagnosis. With a temperature of 103°F or more, a child will usually look and feel terrible, whether the fever is caused by a cold or a serious infection. After the fever is brought down, the child with a cold will look and feel noticeably better—a strong indication that it was the fever itself that was causing the child to look and feel ill—whereas the child with a serious infection will continue to look and feel sick, even with a lower temperature.

In some cases, a feverish child may have what is called a febrile seizure. Febrile seizures, which occur in a very small percentage of children, are frightening to see. They do not seem to be related to the height of the fever or to the rapidity with which it rises, but rather to the idiosyncratic predisposition of certain children. About 50 percent of the children who suffer one febrile seizure will go on to have another one. About 33 percent will have a third one. If your child experiences a febrile seizure, there is a good chance that he could have another.

Although seeing your child experience a seizure is distressing, there is no evidence that febrile seizures cause any permanent harm, nor that this type of convulsion leads to epilepsy or any other seizure disorder. However, if your child has a febrile seizure, it is important to have your doctor examine him to rule out any underlying condition and discuss what to do to prevent a recurrence.

Some children run a fever after a day at an amusement park. Others develop a fever only in response to a serious illness. Your observation of your child's overall condition is the best indicator of its severity. If you are uneasy about your child's condition, call your health care provider for advice.

TAKING YOUR CHILD'S TEMPERATURE

Normal body temperature probably has a much wider range than previously thought. No longer is 98.6°F considered standard. Temperature also varies throughout the day.

In general, any oral temperature over 101°F is considered elevated. However, with the exception of infants less than two months old, it is not usually necessary to treat a temperature under 102°F unless it is making your child uncomfortable.

There are a number of different ways to take a child's temperature: orally, rectally, and under the arm. The way you choose will be determined by your child's age and by her ability to keep still for three minutes or so. In addition to standard mercury thermometers, there are now digital thermometers available that can take a child's temperature in much less time. These are convenient if you have a child who is squirmy and uncomfortable. Another option that is expensive but not as reliable is a device that measures temperature in the ear. If the ear is clogged with wax or the device is not properly positioned in the ear, this type of thermometer will register an inaccurate reading. Another device that measures temperature is the forehead strip. It is the opinion of the authors that these strips are simply not reliable in determining a child's temperature. Ask your nurse or doctor which type or types he or she considers the most reliable.

Regardless of which method you choose, *never* leave any child alone with a thermometer. Also, if you notice a crack in the thermometer, throw it out. The mercury it contains is poisonous.

If your child has just eaten or drunk something warm or cold, is dressed very warmly, or has just been exercising, wait thirty minutes before taking her temperature to be sure you get an accurate reading.

Oral Method

If your child is older than five years, you can take her temperature orally. Wash the thermometer with cool water and then shake it down so that it registers less than 96°F. Place the silver or red end of the thermometer under your child's tongue or alongside her cheek. Either you or your child can hold it in place with your fingers. Don't let your child use her teeth to hold it there. Leave the thermometer in place for three minutes, then remove it.

After reading your child's temperature, wash the thermometer again with cool water and then clean it with isopropyl rubbing alcohol.

Rectal Method

Because young children are so active, and because babies and younger children cannot hold a thermometer in their mouths, a rectal temperature may be your best (or only) option. To take your child's temperature rectally, use a rectal thermometer, which has a round bulb at the end.

Shake down the thermometer so that it registers less than 96°F. Dip the bulb end of the thermometer in petroleum jelly, and insert it about one inch into your baby's rectum. Hold it in place for three minutes, then remove it. It is a good idea to have a towel or washcloth on hand when taking your child's temperature rectally, in case of an "accident" when removing the thermometer.

When reading your child's temperature, be aware that a rectal temperature is usually about 0.8°F higher than an oral temperature. After reading your child's temperature, wash the thermometer with cool water and then clean it with isopropyl rubbing alcohol.

Underarm Method

If your child is less than five years old, or unable to hold a thermometer in her mouth, you can try taking her temperature under the arm. This method usually yields a temperature reading approximately 1°F lower than a child's oral temperature. It also does not always give as reliable a reading as the others do, so it is best used only as a general indicator.

Shake down a standard oral thermometer so that it registers less than 96°F. Place the silver or red end of the thermometer under your child's armpit. Make sure the armpit is dry before placing the thermometer, and leave it in place for three minutes.

After reading your child's temperature, wash the thermometer with cool water and then clean it with isopropyl rubbing alcohol.

EMERGENCY TREATMENT FOR A FEBRILE SEIZURE

Occasionally, a child with a fever will have a seizure. This is called a febrile seizure, and it demands immediate attention.

✚ If your child has a febrile seizure, he needs to see a doctor *immediately*—not tomorrow morning. Call for emergency help.

✚ While waiting for emergency help, keep your child upright and make sure he is breathing well. Stay with him and talk reassuringly to him.

✚ Watch for changes in your child's breathing and/or color. Be sure his airway stays open.

✚ Clear the area around your child to prevent injury. **Do not** try to hold him down. Restraining a thrashing child can cause additional injury. Try placing a soft pillow or blanket under your child's head. Loosen clothing to prevent injury and ease discomfort.

✚ **Do not** try to force anything into your child's mouth to hold down his tongue. You might cause him to choke, or you may suffer a bite yourself.

✚ If vomiting occurs, turn your child's head to the side so that there is no risk of his choking on inhaled vomit. If possible, keep his whole body turned to the side as well.

WHEN TO CALL THE DOCTOR ABOUT A FEVER

There are certain situations in which you should always seek a doctor's advice concerning a child with a fever:

• If your child is under six months of age.

• If your child is between six months and three years old and has a temperature of 102°F or higher.

• If your child is over three years old and has a fever of 105°F or higher that does not respond to normal fever control measures within four hours.

• No matter what your child's age, if he is listless, lethargic, unusually sleepy, in pain, or extremely irritable, or if he complains of a stiff neck, is having difficulty breathing, or has a significant decrease in urine output, or if he just doesn't seem right to you.

• A fever of 106°F or higher is a medical emergency. This child needs immediate medical attention.

GENERAL RECOMMENDATIONS

■ Control measures for conventional fever include giving your child appropriate doses of acetaminophen or ibuprofen (*see* Proper Dosages for Common Over-the-Counter Medications, on page 17).

■ *Do not* give your child aspirin if you suspect she might have a virus.

■ Encourage your child to drink lots of fluids.

■ A warm sponge bath, a tea of lemon balm, chamomile, peppermint, yarrow, and elder flower (either one or a combination of) will help bring down a fever.

■ Certain homeopathics such as *Belladonna* and *Aconite* will help reduce fever.

■ Never sponge your child with cold water or rubbing alcohol.

■ If your child has a febrile seizure, give her a dose of Bach Flower Rescue Remedy while you are waiting for help to arrive or while you are on your way to the doctor's office.

Food Allergies

See also ANAPHYLACTIC REACTION.

An allergy is a hypersensitive reaction to a normally harmless substance. About one in every six children in the United States is allergic to one or more substances. There are a variety of substances, termed allergens, that may trouble your child. Common allergens include pollen, animal dander, house dust, feathers, mites, chemicals, and a variety of foods. This section is devoted to food-related allergies.

Allergic reactions can occur immediately, or they can be delayed and take days to surface. A delayed allergic reaction can make it more difficult to pinpoint the allergen.

Common symptoms of an allergic reaction are respiratory congestion, eye inflammation, swelling, itching, hives, and stomachache and vomiting. Food allergies can contribute to chronic health problems, such as acne, asthma, bedwetting, diarrhea, ear infections, eczema, fatigue, hay fever, headache, irritability, chronic runny nose, and even difficulty maintaining concentration (attention deficit disorder or hyperactivity). Food allergies also can cause intestinal irritation and swelling that interferes with the absorption of vitamins and minerals. Even if you are providing your child with a wholesome, nutritious diet, if she is consuming foods to which she is allergic, she may not be able to absorb food properly, and therefore may not be deriving the full benefits of all the foods she is eating.

The most common foods that cause allergic reactions in children are wheat, milk and other dairy products, eggs, fish and seafood, chocolate, citrus fruits, soy products, corn, nuts, and berries. Many children also are allergic to sulfites, which are found in some frozen foods and dried fruits, as well as in medications. Some people seem to be genetically predisposed to food allergies. If family members, especially parents, have food allergies, there is a greater chance a child will have the same difficulties.

Sometimes, if all the irritating foods are eliminated from a child's diet for several months, her body will have a chance to rest and heal, after which it will be able to handle small amounts of these foods without reacting. Sometimes, too, there is an underlying issue such as a parasitic or yeast infection in the intestine that is contributing to the allergic response. If these underlying problems are cleared up, the child's body may be less reactive to certain substances.

It has been observed that some children actively dislike the foods that produce an allergic reaction. They seem to know instinctively that certain foods will cause a problem. If your child continually refuses particular foods, it may be wise not to force the issue.

Paradoxically, however, some children seem to be particularly drawn to the very foods that cause a problem. For example, many children are sensitive to wheat, a staple in many homes. Children who enthusiastically eat lots of wheat bread, wheat crackers, and wheat cereals, or who crave milk, ice cream, and other dairy products, may actually be exhibiting a sensitivity to those foods.

EMERGENCY TREATMENT FOR FOOD ALLERGIES

✚ Occasionally, an allergic reaction is so severe it can be life threatening. If your child exhibits rapidly spreading hives or has difficulty breathing, seek medical attention immediately.

✚ If there is any sign that your child is having difficulty breathing due to a severe allergic reaction, especially if she has a history of severe reactions, take her immediately to the emergency room of the nearest hospital. If you cannot transport your child yourself, call for emergency help and stress the urgency of the situation. Every second counts.

✚ If an emergency adrenaline kit, such as Ana-Guard, Ana-Kit, or EpiPen, is available, administer it immediately, followed by 25 to 50 milligrams of an antihistamine such as Benadryl. **Do not** give your child anything to eat or drink if she is having difficulty breathing. Even if your child responds quickly to the administration of the emergency adrenaline kit, she should still be taken to the emergency room for professional evaluation and treatment.

GENERAL RECOMMENDATIONS

■ Nutritional supplements, digestive enzymes, and an elimination or rotation diet can be helpful in strengthening a child's body so that it is less susceptible to food allergies. Work closely with a professional health care practitioner.

Food Poisoning

See also DIARRHEA; NAUSEA AND VOMITING.

Food poisoning is most commonly a reaction to toxins produced by bacteria. These organisms thrive in food that is not prepared hygienically, that is kept out of refrigeration for too long, or that is not thoroughly cooked.

Most cases of food poisoning are the result of food being handled by unclean hands or the failure to cook meat long enough and at a high enough temperature to kill microorganisms. For example, if a cook shapes hamburger patties and then cuts raw vegetables, without washing his hands in between, bacteria from the meat can migrate via his hands to contaminate the vegetables. Foods with mayonnaise-type dressings that have been left out of refrigeration for too long can also cause problems, as can cooked foods (such as pizza) that have been removed from heat and left at room temperature for too long. Other food poisonings occur as a result of a toxic reaction to poisonous plants, certain types of mushrooms, or contaminated shellfish. Eating raw fish or shellfish, foods containing raw eggs (such as homemade eggnog or Caesar salad dressing), food that was canned improperly, or food from damaged cans also can lead to food poisoning. Another possible cause is exposure to chemical contaminants such as heavy metals or pesticides.

Common symptoms of food poisoning include nausea, vomiting, diarrhea, abdominal pain and cramping, fever, and general malaise. Symptoms of food poisoning usually come on suddenly, sometimes within hours of eating the contaminated food. Because the symptoms can persist for several days, however, food poisoning is often mistaken for a case of the flu. If your child experiences a sudden bout of nausea, vomiting, and/or diarrhea a couple of hours after eating, he may be suffering from food poisoning.

WHEN TO CALL THE DOCTOR
ABOUT FOOD POISONING

If you have any suspicion of food poisoning, contact your child's physician immediately if any of the following symptoms develop:

- Fever above 102°F.
- Severe vomiting.
- Severe diarrhea, especially if it continues for more than twenty-four hours or contains blood.
- Difficulty breathing or speaking.
- Changes in vision.
- Localized abdominal pain.

Symptoms of Salmonella Poisoning

Salmonella is an increasingly common type of food poisoning. It is the possibility of salmonella contamination that has led to recent recommendations against eating any foods containing raw eggs, for example. Salmonella poisoning usually comes on fairly soon after contact with the contaminated food and runs its course in twenty-four hours or so. Symptoms of salmonella poisoning include:

- Stomach cramps.
- Diarrhea.
- Chills.
- High fever.
- Headache.
- Nausea and vomiting.

Symptoms of Botulism

Botulism is a severe, even potentially life-threatening, form of food poisoning. Any child who displays the symptoms of botulism requires immediate medical attention. Symptoms include:

- Headache and dizziness, beginning sometime between sixteen hours and five days after ingestion of contaminated food.
- Double vision.

- Muscle paralysis.
- Vomiting.
- Difficulty breathing and swallowing.

In babies, symptoms may be:

- Constipation.
- Lethargy.
- Poor muscle tone.

CONVENTIONAL TREATMENT

■ Emetrol, a gentle over-the-counter product, is useful for relieving nausea and vomiting. Follow dosage directions on the product label.

■ For frequent, watery diarrhea, loperamide (Imodium AD) may be helpful. This over-the-counter medication works by slowing the movement of the intestinal muscle. Follow the dosage directions on the product label.

Caution: Do not give loperamide to a child with a fever over 101°F or bloody stools. It is not recommended for children under twelve.

■ If your child's vomiting is severe and he is unable to keep anything down, your doctor may prescribe an antiemetic in suppository form. Prochlorperazine (sold under the brand name Compazine), promethazine (Phenergan), and trimethobenzamide (Tigan) are prescription drugs that are sometimes used for this purpose. Occasionally these are given in injectable form as well.

■ Dimenhydrinate (Dramamine) is sometimes useful for milder vomiting. Follow dosage directions on the product label.

Caution: This medication should not be given to a child under two years old.

■ Activated charcoal, which can be given in capsule form or mixed with water, may be recommended, particularly if a drug or chemical toxin is suspected.

Caution: Do not give charcoal to a child under 8 years old.

GENERAL RECOMMENDATIONS

■ Once the vomiting and/or diarrhea has stopped, give your child an acidophilus or bifidus supplement to help restore healthy flora balance in the intestines.

■ To help ease the vomiting, diarrhea, restlessness, weakness, and burning pain brought on by food poisoning, give your child homeopathic *Arsenicum album* 30c—one dose every two hours, for six hours.

■ The Chinese formula Curing Pills (in liquid form), will help ease most stomach or intestinal upsets.

Fractures

See BONES, BROKEN.

Frostbite

See also HYPOTHERMIA.

Frostbite describes a serious injury to tissue from exposure to very cold temperature. It most commonly affects exposed areas of the body such as the ears, nose, cheeks, and those areas furthest from the heart, such as the fingers and toes. The deeper the frostbite, the more long-term the damage will be to the tissues. Frostbite can be so severe that a person may lose a body part. Any time a child complains of cold, tingling, or numb fingers or toes, take her seriously—bring her inside and immediately warm her up.

You cannot know the extent or degree of the injury until the tissue has been rewarmed. If you suspect your child has frostbite of any body part, take her to your doctor or the nearest emergency room for evaluation and treatment. Depending on the severity of the injury, it may take weeks or months to heal the tissue and regain sensation. There may be a permanent sensitivity to cold in the affected area.

When evaluating frostbite, here's what to look for:

• With *first-degree* frostbite, the skin is numb, red, and slightly swollen.

- With *second-degree* frostbite, the skin begins to blister.
- With *third-degree* frostbite, the blistering is deep.
- With *fourth-degree* frostbite, the damage goes deep into the muscle and may affect the bone.
- A frostbitten area can be cold, pale, and hard. If a large area of the body is affected, such as the entire leg, the area may appear purple rather than white.
- As frostbite gets worse, the pain may actually lessen and eventually disappear as the area becomes numb.

CAUTIONS

■ Do not rub a frostbitten area.

■ Do not attempt to rewarm an area if there is any risk of it getting cold again.

■ Do not allow a child to use a frostbitten body part until it has been treated. For instance, if toes have been frostbitten, do not allow the child to walk until a doctor has evaluated and treated the child.

■ Do not put bandages or salves on the frostbitten area until it has been rewarmed and evaluated by a doctor.

■ When rewarming, use warm water—not hot. Hot water can cause further damage to the injured tissue.

CONVENTIONAL TREATMENT

■ Treatment for frostbite involves rewarming the affected body part in a bath of warm water. This should be done under medical supervision to be sure the water temperature is correct and consistent. This rewarming process is done until the area regains color and softness. It can be a very painful process requiring pain medication such as aspirin, codeine, or morphine.

■ An antibiotic may be prescribed to prevent infection.

■ A severe case of frostbite may need to be treated in a burn center, especially if there is blistering.

GENERAL RECOMMENDATIONS

■ While on the way to the doctor, wrap your child in a blanket to keep her warm, raise the affected limb, and protect it from any further trauma or possible irritation.

■ If blisters develop, do not rupture them. Any open wound is a possible site of infection.

■ For mild cases of frostbite, applying aloe vera gel or cream to the area will be soothing and healing.

PREVENTION

■ Be sure that on cold days your child dresses warmly and in layers. A sweater, vest, or coat are important to keep the trunk warm. If the center of the body is cold, the blood vessels in the hands and feet will narrow so that less blood goes to the extremities while more blood goes to the vital organs.

■ Keeping your child warm and preventing any impairment of circulation are essential in helping to prevent frostbite.

Head Injury

See CONCUSSION.

Headache

Headaches can be caused by muscle tension, an underlying illness or infection, or disturbances in the blood vessels in the head. The latter scenario produces migraine headaches, which typically recur periodically and are characterized by severe pain, often concentrated on one side of the head, that is aggravated by light, sometimes preceded by disturbances in vision, and is often associated with nausea and vomiting. Headaches can sometimes be related to disorders that warrant further investigation, such as infections of the scalp, ears, sinuses, or spinal fluid.

They can also be caused by allergies, fever, high blood pressure, epilepsy, brain tumors, severe tooth cavities or oral infections, certain drugs, or an injury to the head.

Most often, headaches are related to tension. However, if your child awakens crying and holding his head, the cause is most likely something other than tension. If your child has a headache in combination with a high fever, severe vomiting, a stiff neck, confusion, disorientation, or extreme fatigue, see your doctor immediately. This can be a sign of a serious illness, such as meningitis or encephalitis. If a child's headache is so severe that he isn't tempted by a promise of his favorite activity or a favorite food, or if the headaches are frequent and chronic, you should consult with a physician.

A young child with a limited vocabulary may be unable to describe how his head feels. A tension headache often feels like a tight band around the head. The pain may be throbbing or dull, mild or severe. Sudden movements often seem to make a tension headache worse. A headache may develop suddenly or come on gradually. Tension headaches most often develop during the day, worsen as the day goes on, and may be relieved with sleep.

An attack of migraine, on the other hand, can last for days; sleep may or may not be helpful in easing the pain. Some children with migraines may not even complain of head pain, but rather of nausea, vomiting, and stomachache. Migraines can be triggered by a number of different factors, including emotional stress, hypoglycemia, food allergies, head injuries, oral contraceptives, or hormonal changes related to the menstrual cycle, which may be why more females than males suffer from them. The disorder also tends to run in families.

WHEN TO CALL THE DOCTOR ABOUT A HEADACHE

• If your child has a headache in combination with a high fever, extreme fatigue, a stiff neck, severe vomiting, or confusion or disorientation, call your doctor immediately or take your child to the emergency room of the nearest hospital. These can be signs of an infection affecting the brain, such as encephalitis or meningitis.

• If your child's headaches are so severe that they interfere with normal activities, or if they are frequent rather than isolated occurrences, consult with your doctor.

CONVENTIONAL TREATMENT

■ A mild pain reliever, such as ibuprofen (found in Advil, Nuprin, and other medications) or acetaminophen (Tylenol, Tempra, and others) can relieve a headache. These drugs are most effective when given early; headache pain becomes increasingly difficult to relieve as it becomes more severe. Ibuprofen generally works better for headaches, especially migraine headaches, than acetaminophen does.

Caution: Ibuprofen is best given with food to avoid possible stomach upset. Acetaminophen can cause liver damage if taken in excessive amounts. If you give your child acetaminophen, make sure to read package directions carefully so as not to exceed the proper dosage for your child's age and size. (*See* Proper Dosages for Common Over-the-Counter Medications on page 17.)

■ *Do not* give a child aspirin for a headache unless a viral illness has been ruled out by your doctor. The combination of aspirin and certain viral infections is associated with the development of Reye's syndrome, a dangerous liver disease.

■ For extremely severe headaches, a combination of acetaminophen and codeine may be prescribed. Codeine is a powerful narcotic pain-killer that can cause serious side effects, including nausea, sleepiness, and constipation, and that can also be highly addictive.

■ If your child suffers from migraines, ibuprofen or acetaminophen is likely to be suggested first, and may be all that is needed to ease the pain. The antihistamine diphenhydramine (Benadryl) may also be suggested. The reason it works is not well understood, but it may offer relief for your child.

■ A relatively new drug, sumatriptan (sold under the brand name Imitrex), appears to be very effective in alleviating a severe attack of migraine. It works by increasing the amount of serotonin in the brain. Serotonin is involved in vasoconstriction (the constriction of blood vessels); since migraine is in part a result of a disturbance in the brain's blood circulation, increasing serotonin levels may help to restore balance in the tension of blood vessels. This treatment is expensive. It can also produce unpleasant side effects, including increased heart rate, elevated blood pressure, and a feeling of tightness in the chest, jaw, or neck. This drug is not yet officially indicated for use in children.

■ There is some evidence that a daily low dose of beta-blockers such as propranolol (Inderal) may help if a child suffers from recurrent, incapacitating migraine headaches. This drug should not be taken by a child with asthma or diabetes; it can cause such side effects as fatigue, depression, shortness of breath, and cold hands and feet.

■ If your child's headaches are chronic and debilitating, it may be helpful to consult a pediatric neurologist to investigate the possibility of an underlying problem.

GENERAL RECOMMENDATIONS

■ Proper nutrition, homeopathic and herbal treatments, and acupressure can be helpful in their treatment of most headaches, depending on their cause.

■ Massaging the neck, shoulders, and back, taking a warm bath, and drinking a cup of peppermint or chamomile tea can help ease a tension headache.

■ The herb feverfew can be helpful in preventing migraine headaches. It must be taken daily and may take a few months to be effective.

Heat Illness

Heat illness is related to a loss of body fluids and an imbalance in electrolytes caused by exposure to heat. The body may lose its ability to control its heat centers if the heat illness progresses. Children are much more likely to be adversely affected by activity in the heat and sun than adults. Babies and newborns are particularly vulnerable to the heat.

Heat illness is more likely to occur when the air temperature is high and there is relatively high humidity. Playing a physically vigorous sport for hours outside on a hot, humid day without drinking adequate fluids is the perfect setup for heat illness to occur. Early signs of heat illness include red cheeks, muscle weakness, mild confusion, headache, and nausea. A child may feel dizzy and faint. Vomiting is common. A child may or may not sweat.

EMERGENCY TREATMENT
FOR HEAT ILLNESS

✚ A child who has been in the hot sun and is listless, dehydrated, unresponsive, or who is getting sicker despite being out of the heat should be taken to a hospital emergency room and evaluated by medical professionals. Once at the hospital, the child's temperature and overall status will be assessed and continually evaluated until the child is stable.

✚ Intravenous fluids may be administered at the hospital, and measures such as a cool bath or cooling blanket may be used to bring the child's temperature into a normal range.

GENERAL RECOMMENDATIONS

The following recommendations are for cases of mild heat illness.

■ Remove your child from the heat. Place him in a shaded, cooler outdoor area or put him inside a cool room.

■ A child with mild dizziness or weakness should lie down with his feet raised.

■ Remove any heavy clothing from your child and dress him in light, dry clothes. Place him near a fan or sprinkle him with cool water. You can also place cool packs under his arms, at the groin area, or around his neck.

■ Encourage your child to drink as much as possible, especially electrolyte-replacement drinks such as Gatorade or Recharge.

■ A child who has experienced a mild case of heat illness should rest at home for the remainder of the day. There should be no more vigorous activity and certainly no more exposure to the sun or heat.

■ Once treatment has been given and the crisis is over, give your child Bach Flower Rescue Remedy—three drops, three times a day, for one day. Rescue Remedy will help ease any fear, panic, anxiety, or tension. For cases of mild heat illness, your child should not feel sick longer than one day.

■ In addition to Rescue Remedy, give your child homeopathic *Gelsemium* 30c—one dose, three times a day, for one day. *Gelsemium* will help ease any feelings of exhaustion, heaviness, and achiness.

PREVENTION

■ Be sure to dress your child in appropriate clothing on hot days. Have your child wear a sun-hat and loose-fitting, lightweight clothes made of a "breathable" material such as cotton. Change wet clothes.

■ Be sure your child takes periodic breaks from playing in the intense heat and sun to rest in the shade.

■ Be sure your child drinks plenty of fluids with electrolytes on hot days. Don't wait until your child stops playing to offer him drinks—rather offer him fluids throughout the day. Citrus juice, Gatorade, and Recharge are good choices.

■ Be sure your child eats nourishing meals throughout the day.

Hemorrhage

See BLEEDING, SEVERE.

Hypothermia

See also FROSTBITE.

Hypothermia—abnormally low body temperature (below 95°F or 35°C)—is the result of prolonged exposure to cold air or water. This is a serious condition that can be life threatening or cause severe damage to the muscular and nervous systems. A decrease in core temperature can occur on very cold days, as well as cool summer days, if a child is in cold, wet clothes for hours and cannot warm up. A child who is tired, hungry, dehydrated, or sick may develop hypothermia even if the outside temperature is not that cold.

Mild hypothermia can begin with feelings of persistent chilliness and skin numbness with some mental confusion and change in muscle coordination. As hypothermia progresses, the child typically becomes more uncoordinated, unable to walk, confused, lethargic, and irrational. In severe hypothermia, the child becomes unconscious and rigid with dramatically slowed breathing and heart rate.

EMERGENCY TREATMENT FOR HYPOTHERMIA

✚ If a child has progressed into severe hypothermia, he must be taken to the nearest emergency room. While on the way, try not to let the child get any colder, but do not actually try to rewarm him. (Do not assume that a situation is hopeless until the child has been rewarmed by qualified professionals. The heart rate may be so slow that it may only appear to have stopped.)

✚ In an outdoor situation, the best treatment is direct skin contact with another person. Remove the child's clothing and place him between two unclothed people underneath a blanket or in a sleeping bag.

CONVENTIONAL TREATMENT

The following methods are for treating mild cases of hypothermia.

■ First, it is important to be aware of the problem. When your child complains of being cold or you notice that he is shivering, bring him into the warmth immediately.

■ Dress your child in more clothing—especially cover his head and neck. Replace wet clothing with dry.

■ Have your child drink lots of warm liquids.

■ In order to increase the body's heat production, have your child engage in some physical activity, such as running in place, swinging his arms around, and jumping up and down.

GENERAL RECOMMENDATIONS

■ For mild hypothermia, have your child sip a cup of warm ginger tea.

■ Keep a thermometer handy when camping with children.

PREVENTION

■ When playing outdoors on a cold day, your child should be dressed warmly and in layers. Do not let him wear any constricting clothing. Be sure he wears a hat and gloves or mittens.

■ Be sure your child is well-hydrated when playing outdoors in the cold. Give him lots of fluids throughout the day—don't rely on him to tell you he is thirsty.

■ Be sure your child eats well and often on cold days.

■ Remove wet clothes immediately.

Insect Bites

See BITES AND STINGS, INSECT.

Lyme Disease

See under BITES AND STINGS, INSECT.

Meningitis

Meningitis is an infection and inflammation of the three *meninges*, the thin membranes that cover the brain and spinal cord. The infection can be caused by either a virus or bacteria. *Hemophilus influenzae,* or "H. flu.," is the most common among the bacterial organisms that cause meningitis in children. An infection in the blood (bacteremia), ears, jaws, or sinuses can also lead to an infection of the meninges.

A newborn with meningitis may have poor muscle tone, difficulty feeding, a weak suck and cry, vomiting, irritability, sleepiness and/or jitteriness. In infants, symptoms of meningitis include a high-pitched cry, irritability, loss of appetite, vomiting, lethargy, a bulging or tight fontanel (soft spot), and possibly a fever or convulsions. An older child is likely to have fever, chills, vomiting, irritability, headache, and /or a stiff neck. Seizures and changes in consciousness, such as stupor or coma, are possible as the infection progresses.

Meningitis is a serious infection that is potentially life threatening and can cause such long-term consequences as hearing or vision problems. It requires immediate medical attention. If your child displays any of the symptoms described above, particularly after or while recovering from a respiratory illness or sore throat, call your doctor right away. If treated early and appropriately, there is a low likelihood of complications or lasting harm to your child.

CONVENTIONAL TREATMENT

◼ Meningitis is diagnosed by looking for signs of infection and the presence of an infectious organism in the spinal fluid. To perform a "spinal tap," a needle is inserted into a space between two vertebrae and a small amount of fluid is withdrawn for inspection. The process can be difficult, as it requires the child to curl up and lie still. The doctor will use a numbing medicine on the skin before putting in the needle to lessen the pain, but it still feels like pressure in the back. The doctor will probably also take a sample of your child's blood to look for other signs of infection.

◼ If meningitis is suspected, antibiotic therapy will be started immediately after spinal fluid samples are taken. A doctor will not wait to get the results back to find out whether the meningitis is bacterial or viral, because the risks of not treating a possible bacterial infection immediately are too great. The antibiotic will be given intravenously, usually for a minimum of seven days. Ampicillin, penicillin, and chloramphenicol are commonly used antibiotics for bacterial meningitis.

◼ If the meningitis is determined to be viral in origin, antibiotics are ineffective and will be discontinued. Rest, fluids, and nutritious foods, as well as measures to control fever and relieve pain, will be recommended to ease the discomfort and aid in recovery.

◼ If there is *even a suspicion* of viral meningitis, aspirin should not be given, because the combination of aspirin and viral infection has been linked to the development of Reyes Syndrome, a dangerous disease affecting the brain and liver.

GENERAL RECOMMENDATIONS

■ During the acute phase of meningitis, a quiet, dimly lit room will help ease the headache pain. Stories, a soothing massage, and holding your child, will help reassure him and ease his discomfort.

■ If your child contracts bacterial meningitis, be aware of the possibility of subtle injury to the brain. Don't hesitate to talk to your doctor if you are worried about persistent hearing loss, problems with balance or coordination, difficulties with schoolwork, or similar difficulties.

■ Once the infection has been resolved, give your child small amounts of American ginseng for one month to help nourish and strengthen his system. Also give your child a daily multivitamin and mineral supplement.

■ Give your child an acidophilus or bifidus supplement to help restore a healthy balance of intestinal flora.

PREVENTION

■ Most medical doctors now recommend that children be routinely given the Hib vaccine, which offers immunity against *Hemophilus influenzae* bacteria (the most common cause of bacterial meningitis), starting when they are two months of age. This can be given either by itself or in combination with the DPT vaccine.

Nail Injuries

Injuries to the fingernails and toenails are common in childhood. Children are curious, and their hands seem to get into everything. Little fingers and car doors sometimes come together with disastrous results. Splinters find their way underneath fingernails. A badly caught ball can jam a finger and injure a nail. Rocks can get dropped, and bare toes often get stubbed.

Depending on the extent and type of injury, a bruise may form immediately. The area may appear red and swollen, or white and scraped. More seriously, a nail can be completely torn off.

Any injury to tissue makes infection a possibility. If a nail injury does not improve within twenty-four hours, or if the area begins to show increasing redness, warmth, swelling, or other signs of infection, call your physician.

EMERGENCY TREATMENT FOR NAIL INJURIES

✚ If there is intense pain and pressure after a nail injury, it is possible that a "blood blister" is forming underneath the nail that may need to be drained. See your health care provider or take your child to a hospital emergency room for evaluation and care. If necessary, a doctor can relieve the pressure by making a small hole in the nail so that the blood can drain. This may also be an opportunity to update your child's tetanus vaccination, if necessary.

GENERAL RECOMMENDATIONS

■ Cleanse the area with cold water.

■ If the nail has been partially torn from the finger or toe, bandage it lightly with the remaining nail held loosely in place. Keep the area protected against further injury with a small splint or finger cup.

■ If part of the nail bed is exposed, or if there is an open wound, apply an antibiotic or calendula ointment before bandaging. Keep the area bandaged until the injury heals.

■ Once proper medical attention has been given, a number of homeopathic remedies will help speed healing and ease pain and swelling. On day one, give your child *Arnica* 30x, three times. On day two, give her *Ledum* 30x, three times. And on days three and four, give her *Hypericum* 12x, three times each day.

Nausea and Vomiting

Symptoms of stomach upset may begin with loss of appetite, proceed to queasiness or nausea, then actual pain—either constant or crampy—

in the upper stomach, followed by vomiting and, occasionally, diarrhea. A child may complain of a "headache in my stomach," or an abdomen that feels "full" or crampy. The pain may be in one spot, all over the abdomen, or travel around. The abdomen may be tender to the touch. Vomiting may occur, perhaps with waves of nausea right before an episode and temporary relief afterwards.

Childhood stomachaches have a wide variety of physical and emotional causes. In an infant, a stomachache and vomiting can be associated with serious problems, including meningitis, urinary tract infection, feeding difficulties, and anatomical defects. In older children, a stomachache and vomiting can be the result of food poisoning, overeating, motion sickness, infection, hepatitis, appendicitis, constipation, meningitis, muscle strain, tiredness, food allergies, or the accidental ingestion of drugs and poisons. Emotional upsets, such as homesickness, sorrow, nervousness, anger, or anticipation of an upcoming event, can translate into stomach upsets. A child wrestling with feelings surrounding divorce, a new sibling, holidays, a final exam, or school phobia can develop a stomachache.

A single episode of nausea or vomiting is likely to be a reaction to some food your child has eaten, or a sign of emotional upset. When nausea is severe or persists for more than a few hours, the most likely cause is either food poisoning or an infection. Bacterial infections can be caused by a wide variety of organisms, including *Campylobacter*, *Escherichia coli* (E. coli), *Salmonella*, *Shigella*, or *Staphylococcus*. Vomiting related to a bacterial infection of the intestine often will be accompanied by diarrhea and fever, whereas food poisoning caused by a bacterial toxin is less likely to cause a fever. Viral infections can also cause diarrhea. By listening to your child's history and symptoms, and by performing tests and a physical examination, your doctor can help diagnose the underlying cause of your child's stomachache and/or vomiting so that you can treat the illness properly.

If an underlying illness has been ruled out and your child is still complaining of a stomachache, you might want to consider emotional causes for his distress. Talking to your child and to your child's doctor, teachers, school counselors, or even a child therapist can be a good place to start. Keep in mind that even if your child's symptoms are emotional in origin, the discomfort they cause is real and they deserve treatment and attention, just as they would if they were physically based.

WHEN TO CALL THE DOCTOR
ABOUT NAUSEA AND VOMITING

• If your child has projectile vomiting—a violent episode in which the vomit is ejected in a forceful stream and lands at a distance from his mouth—call your doctor right away. This can be an indication of a serious problem.

• If your child experiences nausea and vomiting with progressive pain and tenderness in the lower right abdomen, seek medical help immediately. It may signify the development of appendicitis. Typically, appendicitis pain starts around the umbilicus and gradually travels to and localizes around the lower right-hand quadrant of the abdomen. Appendicitis is often associated with a fever. (See APPENDICITIS.)

• If your child experiences any of the following, consult your physician: persistent vomiting; blood in the vomit; abdominal pain so severe that it keeps your child from eating, playing, or other normal activities; persistent abdominal pain that lasts more than a few hours.

CONVENTIONAL TREATMENT

■ Your child's doctor will perform an examination to determine whether the nausea and vomiting are caused by an infection or toxin, emotional distress, or an internal obstruction. He or she will look for signs of dehydration, fever, abdominal tenderness, or blood in the stool. If diarrhea is present, a stool culture may help to determine if the vomiting is related to a bacterial infection. Your doctor will recommend treatment based on the likely cause of your child's distress.

■ Antiemetics are drugs that are sometimes prescribed to ease nausea and stop vomiting. Trimethobenzamide (Tigan), prochlorperazine (Compazine), and promethazine (Phenergan) are among the ones most commonly used. They can be given in tablet or suppository form, or by injection. Because these drugs can have serious side effects, they should be used with caution in children. Never administer more than the prescribed dose.

■ Over-the-counter antacids, such as Maalox, Mylanta, and Rolaids, may be helpful for an occasional stomachache caused by acid indigestion or heartburn. Antacids neutralize acidic secretions in the stomach. However, because some antacids can actually end up increasing the production of acids in the stomach, or cause constipation or diarrhea, they are not routinely recommended for children.

■ Emetrol is a safe, over-the-counter syrup that settles the stomach. It is useful for relief of nausea caused by infections, overeating, or emotional upset, and produces no side effects. Give your child the proper dosage as directed on the product label.

■ Bismuth subsalicylate, more commonly known as Pepto-Bismol, absorbs toxins and provides a protective coating along the gastrointestinal tract. It is helpful for relief of nausea as well as of diarrhea.

■ Unless specifically prescribed by your doctor, **do not** give a child with a stomachache a pain reliever, such as acetaminophen, aspirin, or ibuprofen. In relieving stomach pain whose cause has not been diagnosed, you may be masking an underlying condition that could become worse without treatment.

GENERAL RECOMMENDATIONS

■ Ginger, peppermint, or chamomile tea may help relieve nausea.

■ To help relieve persistent or incessant nausea and vomiting, give your child one dose of homeopathic *Ipecac* 12x or 6c every hour, up to four doses.

Neck Injury

See BONES, BROKEN.

Nosebleed

There are a great many tiny blood vessels in the delicate lining of the nose. These small capillaries are easily broken. Any number of things can rupture some of these small vessels and cause a nosebleed.

A fall from a jungle gym or bicycle, or a swat from an angry playmate or sibling, may cause a child's nose to bleed. If your child suffers a bloody nose from one of these causes, expect some hollering. A blow to the nose can be very painful.

If your child puts something in her nose, a nosebleed can occur. Even just blowing the nose can start one. Inflammation from a cold, an allergy, even dry winter air, can cause the vessels to swell and rupture. Your child may awaken with blood on her sheets or nightclothes. When a nosebleed from one of these causes occurs, it seldom hurts.

Blood can be swallowed during a nosebleed, especially one that occurs during the night. If enough blood is involved, your child may vomit it up, or pass a dark, tarry-looking stool after the nosebleed has stopped.

The amount of blood coming from the nose during a nosebleed can be a continuous stream or just a small trickle. It may look as if your child is losing a lot of blood, but not much blood is actually lost during the typical nosebleed. Although a bloody nose can be frightening to a child, it can usually be managed easily at home. Like most wounds, ruptured capillaries inside the nose will heal in about ten days.

If your child has a medical condition that makes her prone to nose-bleeds, such as high blood pressure, leukemia, or hemophilia, ask your doctor for advice. If your child's nosebleeds recur more than once a month or so, have her examined by a doctor to rule out a possible underlying cause.

HOW TO STOP A NOSEBLEED

✚ To stop the bleeding, apply pressure to the bridge of your child's nose, as follows:

1. Sit your child upright and tilt her head forward (*not* backward).

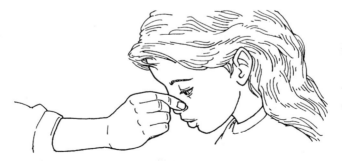

2. Place your thumb and forefinger on either side of the bridge of the nose (*see* above). And apply pressure firmly enough to slow bleeding, but not so strongly as to cause discomfort. Pressure decreases the blood flow through the affected area, slowing bleeding. To give a clot time to form, maintain the pressure for about ten minutes.

3. After ten minutes, check to see if the bleeding has stopped. If not, apply pressure for another ten-minute period.

4. If your child's nose is still bleeding steadily after twenty minutes of pressure, call your doctor.

✚ You can also place an ice pack across the bridge of your child's nose. This will constrict the blood vessels and help stop the bleeding. Hold the ice pack firmly in place. After ten minutes, check to see if bleeding has stopped. If not, reapply the ice pack for another ten-minute period. If your child's nose is still bleeding steadily after twenty minutes, call your doctor.

CONVENTIONAL TREATMENT

■ In the event of a severe nosebleed, your doctor may pack your child's nose with gauze, and instruct you to leave the packing in place for one or two days.

■ For an exceptionally serious nosebleed, your physician may recommend cauterizing the broken blood vessels within the nose. This involves applying an electrical current or silver nitrate stick directly to the broken vessel to solidify blood at the site. In very rare cases of severe, recurrent nosebleeds, a surgical tie-off of one of the larger blood vessels that supplies the tiny capillaries in the lining of the nose is recommended. Fortunately, this procedure is rarely necessary.

GENERAL RECOMMENDATIONS

■ Humidify the air in your home, especially the bedrooms. This will help keep the inner lining of the nose moist and lessen the chance of small capillaries from swelling and rupturing.

■ Before bedtime, apply a small amount of bacitracin ointment to the nasal septum (the inner wall of the nose) to keep the area moist.

■ To help resolve a nosebleed and speed healing of the injured tissue, give your child one dose of homeopathic *Ferrum phosphoricum* 6x or 12x, every ten minutes for a total of four doses.

Overdose, Drug

See POISONING.

Poison Ivy, Oak, and Sumac

The rash associated with a case of poison ivy, oak, or sumac is an allergic reaction to a resin contained in the leaves, stems, and roots of these poisonous plants. Because these plants are most abundant during the spring, most cases occur at that time of the year.

The rash and treatment of these three conditions are similar. This entry focuses mainly on poison ivy, the most common of the three, but what is true for poison ivy is true also for poison oak and poison sumac.

A child can get poison ivy from the plant itself or by touching anything that has come in contact with the plant and has some of the resinous oil on it. For example, if a child picks up a rake that has been resting in a bed of poison ivy, the characteristic rash may develop. If clothing or the part of the body that touched the plant is not carefully washed, the oil can be spread to other parts of the body, or even be transmitted to another person. Another, and potentially quite serious, form of exposure can occur through the inhalation of smoke from burning leaves if there are parts of the poison ivy plant among them.

A poison ivy rash can appear anywhere from a few hours to a few days after contact with the resin. The rash can last from one to four weeks, and is usually at its worst four to seven days after exposure. The severity of the condition depends on the amount of contact with the resinous oil, as well as how sensitive the child is to the plant. Not everyone is allergic to poison ivy. The resin may not bother some children at all, while others develop a serious and extensive rash.

The rash first appears as red, very itchy pimples that may develop into small fluid-filled blisters. If the contact occurred with the edge of a leaf, the eruption may form in a straight line. As with all skin rashes and wounds, it is possible for the area to become infected. If you notice signs of local infection, such as increased redness, swelling, or warmth or tenderness at the site, seek medical advice.

If your child experiences pain or swelling on the face or genitals and is uncomfortable because of this, or if the rash is very extensive, medical care may be warranted. Otherwise, most cases of poison ivy can be treated successfully at home.

WHEN TO CALL THE DOCTOR
ABOUT POISON IVY, OAK, OR SUMAC

• If there is any sign that your child is developing difficulty breathing as a result of an allergic reaction to poison ivy, oak, or sumac, seek emergency medical treatment.

• If your child experiences pain or swelling on the face or genitals, or if the rash is very extensive and/or causing extreme discomfort, call your doctor.

• As with any skin disorder, it is possible for an area affected by poison ivy, oak, or sumac to become infected. If you notice signs of a developing local infection, such as increased redness, swelling, warmth, or tenderness at the site, consult your physician.

CONVENTIONAL TREATMENT

■ Calamine lotion is an old standby that temporarily eases the itching of poison ivy. However, if used for more than one week, calamine lotion can harden and dry the skin, causing more problems. Caladryl is a combination lotion of calamine and benadryl that may be helpful in relieving the itching.

■ Rhulicream and Rhuligel are over-the-counter preparations that may be more effective than calamine at relieving the itching of poison ivy. Follow the application directions on the product label.

■ Benadryl and Chlor-Trimeton are two over-the-counter oral antihistamines that can help with the itching and swelling of poison ivy.

■ In severe cases, an oral or topical steroid, such as prednisone, may be prescribed to lessen itching and especially to decrease inflammation. Steroids are strong and work quickly, but because of potential side effects, they are not suitable for long-term use and are generally reserved for very serious cases. Also, if steroids are stopped too soon or too

Recognizing Poison Ivy, Oak, and Sumac

The best way to prevent a bout with poison ivy, poison oak, or poison sumac is to know how to recognize these plants and avoid them.

Poison ivy (*Rhus radicans*), by far the most common of the three, is usually thought of as a vine, but it can also grow straight up, like a shrub, to a height of anywhere between two and seven feet. It grows equally happily in woods, partly wooded areas and thickets, and suburban back yards, and can be found virtually anywhere in the United States and southern Canada. Its leaves are often shiny bright green, but not always; the edges can be smooth or jagged. In the fall, the leaves can turn a brilliant bronze-red, and drooping clusters of white berries appear. The distinctive feature of poison ivy, and the thing to look for, is that its leaves always occur in groups of three, with the end leaflet pointed and on a slightly longer stalk than the side pair. If you see any plant whose leaves match this description, avoid it and warn your child to stay well away from it. Touching any part of the poison ivy plant is dangerous.

Poison oak (*Rhus toxicodendron*) is similar to poison ivy in most respects. The only important differences to note are that this plant always grows in shrub form, and that the leaves, while still occurring in trios, are shaped more like oak leaves.

Poison sumac (*Rhus vernix*) is less common than poison ivy or poison oak, which is a good thing, because it is much more toxic. Touching any part of the plant can result in a severe rash and allergic reaction. The poison sumac plant, which is found primarily in swampy, partly wooded areas in the eastern half of the United States and Canada, takes the form of a shrub or small tree with leaves consisting of seven to thirteen (but always an odd number) pointed leaflets. The edges of the leaflets are smooth, not jagged. From late summer to early spring, the plant has whitish berries that occur in clusters.

If your child does come into contact with any of these plants, you should take measures immediately to wash off the resin with either soap and water or jewelweed juice (*see* General Recommendations, this entry).

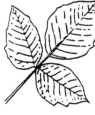
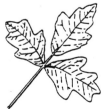
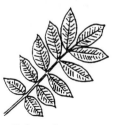

Poison Ivy   Poison Oak   Poison Sumac

abruptly, the rash may get worse as a result of a "rebound" effect. It is wise to use steroids in only the most extreme situations.

■ Cold compresses applied for twenty minutes every few hours are useful for soothing and decreasing the swelling.

■ If the rash is inflamed, red, and oozing, Burow's solution may help. This over-the-counter product is both astringent and antiseptic, but it is mild on the skin. It may be diluted even further than the label directions indicate if it seems to irritate your child's skin.

■ Aloe vera gel can be very helpful in decreasing inflammation. It is best to use fresh gel from a plant or a commercial product with a high concentration of aloe vera.

GENERAL RECOMMENDATIONS

■ After known exposure to poison ivy, thoroughly wash the area of contact with soap and water as soon as possible. Because unexposed areas of skin may come in contact with the oil as clothing is stripped off, a thorough shower is probably the best way to make sure all of the resin is washed off. If no washing facilities are available, do what you can to cleanse the area that made contact with the plant. Change clothes as soon as possible, taking care to avoid contact with contaminated areas. Washing or rinsing with grindelia juice may also be helpful. The resinous oil of poison ivy penetrates the skin in about ten minutes. After ten minutes, it cannot be washed off.

■ Soak a clean cotton cloth in a blend of 1 tablespoon sea salt dissolved in one pint of spring water. To relieve itching, apply the compress to the affected area for fifteen to thirty minutes several times daily.

■ Cold cucumber slices applied to the affected area can help dry out an oozing rash.

■ Clothing that has come in contact with the oil should be washed in a strong detergent with chlorine bleach added.

■ *Rhus toxicodendron*—homeopathic poison ivy—will help relieve itching quickly. Give your child one dose of *Rhus toxicodendron* 12x or 6c, three to four times a day, until symptoms lessen.

150

Poisoning

See also FOOD POISONING.

Eighty percent of all poisonings occur in children under five years old. Small children use their mouths to learn about the world. Anyone who has watched an infant knows that everything—clothes, toes, fingers, toys—goes into a baby's mouth.

Accidental poisonings in childhood most often occur as a result of ingesting harmful substances found around the home. In the 1980s, the Environmental Protection Agency reported that there were over 58,000 chemical substances available in the United States. Since new products are being created all the time, we can safely assume that there are now considerably more than that. Medicines, cleaning products, paints, varnishes, pesticides, hobby supplies, and cosmetics all contain harmful chemicals. Worse, these products are often packaged in bright and attractive colors that catch the eye of an exploring child. The chemicals they contain can cause serious injury or even death if a child ingests them.

Another type of childhood poisoning occurs as a result of a child receiving too much medication or an incorrect medication. This can happen if a child is given a prescription originally written for another person. To share medications is to risk the possibility that your child may receive a toxic dose of a drug. Vitamin tablets, especially those with iron, are a common source of overdose.

Some common houseplants and outdoor plants are poisonous. A number of children are poisoned every year by ingesting a toxic leaf, flower, or berry from a plant.

Although most children who ingest poisons are very young, the incidence of poisonings among adolescents is on the rise in the United States. The adolescent who ingests a toxic or poisonous substance may be making a suicide gesture, which must be taken seriously. An adolescent who intentionally takes an overdose of a toxic substance may be seeking attention or adventure, or may seriously wish to end her life. Adolescents can also get into trouble by experimenting with or overdosing on street drugs. Once the immediate crisis has been handled, professional counseling is crucial for both child and parents to determine and deal with the deeper issues involved.

EMERGENCY TREATMENT
FOR POISONING

A child who has ingested a poisonous substance needs emergency treatment. However, proper treatment depends on the nature of the poison involved. If you know that your child has ingested a poisonous substance, follow the appropriate steps outlined below. If you are not certain about the nature of the poison, call your local Poison Control Center and ask for advice. For a list of Poison Control Centers in the United States and Canada, *see* page 155.

✚ If your child has ingested a noncaustic, nonpetroleum-based product, such as a medication, street drug, or a poisonous plant:

1. Immediately remove any toxic substances visible in your child's mouth.

2. Call the local Poison Control Center at once for information on what steps to take. Try to remain calm, and be as specific as possible in describing your child's age and weight, the possible source of the poisoning, the amount of poison ingested, and the time elapsed. Poison Control may tell you to administer syrup of ipecac to induce vomiting, and then to call an ambulance or take your child to the emergency room of the nearest hospital.

3. Administer ipecac according to the directions given by the Poison Control Center (*see* Administering Syrup of Ipecac on page 153).
   Caution: Do not give syrup of ipecac to a child less than one year old or to a child who is unconscious, who has a history of heart disease, or whose gag reflex may not be working properly.

4. After your child has vomited, take her at once to the emergency room. Take the bottle or package of suspect material with you. It may save valuable time in determining what treatment is necessary.

✚ If your child has ingested a caustic acid or alkali product, such as lye, drain cleaner, oven cleaner, toilet bowl cleaner, electric dishwasher detergent, or swimming pool cleaner:

1. Immediately remove any toxic substances visible in your child's mouth.

2. If a caustic substance is in her eyes or on her skin, immediately flush the area with large amounts of clean running water to prevent damage to the area and absorption into the body.

3. ***Do not induce vomiting.*** Causing a child to vomit after ingestion of caustic substances can cause additional damage to the esophagus and mouth as the substance comes back up.

4. Call the local Poison Control Center at once for information on what steps to take. Try to remain calm, and be as specific as possible in describing your child and identifying the possible source of the poisoning. Poison Control may tell you to dilute the substance in your child's stomach, and then to call an ambulance or take your child to the emergency room of the nearest hospital.

5. To dilute the substance in your child's stomach, give her two glasses of water or milk immediately. Either one will dilute the substance and help to minimize damage.

6. When taking your child to the emergency room, take the bottle or package of suspect material with you. It may save valuable time in determining what treatment is necessary.

✚ **If your child has ingested a petroleum-based product, such as gasoline, oil, turpentine, benzene, kerosene, lighter fluid, furniture polish, moth-balls, or lubricating fluid:**

1. Immediately remove any toxic substances visible in your child's mouth.

2. If a caustic substance is in her eyes or on her skin, immediately flush the area with large amounts of clean running water to prevent damage to the area and absorption into the body.

3. *Do not induce vomiting.* Causing a child to vomit after ingestion of a petroleum-based substance can cause additional damage to the esophagus and mouth as the substance comes back up.

4. Call an ambulance or take your child to the emergency room of the nearest hospital at once. Take the bottle or package of suspect material with you. It may save valuable time in determining what treatment is necessary.

ADMINISTERING SYRUP OF IPECAC

Syrup of ipecac is an over-the-counter drug that usually causes a person to vomit quickly when it is swallowed. In certain cases of poisoning, the best treatment is to get the toxic substance out of the victim's stomach as quickly as possible. Syrup of ipecac is excellent for this.

Sometimes, however, inducing vomiting will do more harm than good. This largely depends on the nature of the poisonous substance ingested. *Do not* use syrup of ipecac if your child has swallowed any of the following:

- Alkalis, such as lye, dishwasher detergent, drain cleaner, oven cleaner, etc.

- Petroleum distillates, such as furniture polish, kerosene, gasoline, oil-based paint, lighter fluid, etc.

If your child has ingested a poisonous substance and your local Poison Control Center advises you to use syrup of ipecac to induce vomiting before taking your child to the emergency room, follow the instructions they give you on how to administer the drug. **Do not** use ipecac unless you are instructed to do so by the Poison Control Center. The amount you will be told to use will depend on your child's size. Generally, if your child weighs 25 pounds or less, the dosage should be 1 tablespoon; if your child weighs over 25 pounds, the dosage should be 2 tablespoons. After your child has swallowed the ipecac, have her drink at least 12 ounces of water to ensure vomiting. Try to keep her walking around. If she has not vomited in twenty minutes, you may be instructed to administer another dose of ipecac, followed by another 12 ounces of water.

Do not give any child more than two doses of ipecac. Do not give a child less than one year old a second dose of ipecac. The vomiting caused by ipecac can be very violent. If the second dose is unsuccessful, abandon the attempt and take your child at once to the emergency room of the nearest hospital.

When your child vomits, have her lie on her side with her mouth lower than her chest, so that the vomited material will not reenter the airway and cause more trouble. If she leans over a toilet to vomit, make sure her chest is lower than her stomach.

There are a number of situations in which syrup of ipecac should *never* be used:

- Never give ipecac to a child less than one year old unless directed to do so by a doctor or the Poison Control Center..

- Never attempt to give ipecac to a child who is unconscious.

- Never give ipecac to a child with a history of heart disease.

- Never give ipecac to a child whose gag reflex may not be working properly, such as a child who has ingested sedatives or tranquilizers, a child who is drowsy, or one who may be drunk.

EMERGENCY POISON CONTROL CENTER TELEPHONE NUMBERS

The following are telephone numbers for local Poison Control Centers in the United States and Canada. In an emergency, call your regional center. Because area codes and phone numbers are subject to change, it is a wise precaution to know the current phone number of your local center and post it near every telephone in your home. If you can program your telephone for automatic dialing, add the number to your phone's programming as well.

ALABAMA

205–939–9201
205–933–4050
800–292–6678 (AL only)

ALASKA

907–261–3193

ARIZONA

Statewide
800–362–0101 (AZ only)

Phoenix Region
602–253–3334

Tucson Region
602–626–6016

ARKANSAS

501–686–6161

CALIFORNIA

Davis Region
916–734–3692
800–342–9293 (No. CA only)

Fresno Region
209–445–1222
800–346–5922 (CA only)

Orange County Region
714–634–5988
800–544–4404 (So. CA only)

San Diego Region
619–543–6000
800–876–4766 (619 area only)

San Francisco/Bay Area
415–476–6600

San Jose/Santa Clara Valley
408–299–5112
800–662–9886 (CA only)

COLORADO

303–629–1123

CONNECTICUT

203–679–1000
800–343–2722 (CT only)

DELAWARE

302–655–3389

DISTRICT OF COLUMBIA

202–625–3333
202–784–4660 (TTY*)

FLORIDA

813–253–4444
800–282–3171 (FL only)

*Teletype, for the hearing-impaired.

GEORGIA
404–589–4400
800–282–5846 (GA only)

HAWAII
808–941–4411

IDAHO
208–378–2707
800–632–8000 (ID only)

ILLINOIS
217–753–3330
800–543–2022 (IL only)
800–942–5969

INDIANA
317–929–2323
800–382–9097 (IN only)

IOWA
800–272–6477 (IA only)
800–362–2327 (IA only)

KANSAS
Topeka/Northern Kansas
913–354–6100

Wichita/Southern Kansas
316–263–9999

KENTUCKY
502–629–7275
800–722–5725 (KY only)

LOUISIANA
800–256–9822 (LA only)

MAINE
800–442–6305 (ME only)

MARYLAND
Statewide
410–528–7701
800–492–2414 (MD only)

D.C. Suburbs
202–625–3333
202–784–4660 (TTY*)

MASSACHUSETTS
617–232–2120
800–682–9211

MICHIGAN
Statewide
800–632–2727 (MI only)
800–356–3232 (TTY*)

Detroit Region
313–745–5711

MINNESOTA
Statewide
800–222–1222

Duluth/Northern Minnesota
218–726–5466

Minneapolis/St. Paul Region
612–347–3141
612–337–7474 (TDD**)
612–221–2113

**Telecommunication device for
the deaf.

MISSISSIPPI
601–354–7660

MISSOURI
314–772–5200
800–366–8888

MONTANA
303–629–1123

NEBRASKA
Statewide
800–955–9119 (NE only)

Omaha Region
402–390–5555

NEVADA
702–732–4989

NEW HAMPSHIRE
603–650–5000
800–562–8236 (NH only)

NEW JERSEY
800–962–1253

NEW MEXICO
505–843–2551
800–432–6866 (NM only)

NEW YORK
Albany Region
800–336–6997

Binghamton/Southern Tier
800–252–5655

Buffalo/Western New York
716–878–7654
800–888–7655

Long Island
516–542–2323
516–542–2324
516–542–2325
516–542–3813

New York City
212–340–4494
212–POISONS
212–689–9014 (TDD**)

Nyack/Hudson Valley
914–353–1000

Syracuse/Central New York
315–476–4766

NORTH CAROLINA
Statewide
800–672–1697

Charlotte Region
704–355–4000

NORTH DAKOTA
800–732–2200 (ND only)

OHIO
Statewide
800–682–7625

Columbus/Central Ohio
614–228–1323
614–461–2012
614–228–2272 (TTY*)

Cincinnati Region
513–558–5111
800–872–5111 (OH only)

OKLAHOMA
800–522–4611 (OK only)

OREGON
503–494–8968
800–452–7165 (OR only)

PENNSYLVANIA
Hershey/Central Pennsylvania
800–521–6110

Philadelphia/E. Pennsylvania
215–386–2100

Pittsburgh/W. Pennsylvania
412–681–6669

PUERTO RICO
809–754–8535

RHODE ISLAND
401–277–5727

SOUTH CAROLINA
803–777–1117

SOUTH DAKOTA
800–952–0123 (SD only)

TENNESSEE
Memphis/Western Tennessee
901–528–6048

Nashville/Eastern Tennessee
615–322–6435

TEXAS
214–590–5000
800–441–0040 (TX only)

UTAH
801–581–2151
800–456–7707 (UT only)

VERMONT
800–562–8236 (VT only)

VIRGINIA
Statewide
800–451–1428

Charlottesville/Blue Ridge
804–925–5543

D.C. Suburbs
202–625–3333
202–784–4660 (TTY*)

WASHINGTON
800–732–6985 (WA only)

WEST VIRGINIA
304–348–4211
800–642–3625 (WV only)

WISCONSIN
**Madison/S.W. and
N. Wisconsin**
608–262–3702

Milwaukee/S.E. Wisconsin
414–266–2222

WYOMING
800–955–9119 (WY only)

CANADA

ALBERTA
403–670–1414

BRITISH COLUMBIA
604–682–5050

MANITOBA
204–787–2591

NEW BRUNSWICK
Fredericton
506–452–5400

Saint John
506–648–6222

NEWFOUNDLAND
709–722–1110

NOVA SCOTIA
902–428–8161

ONTARIO
613–737–1100 (E. Ontario)
800–267–1373 (Ontario only)

PRINCE EDWARD ISLAND
902–428–8161

QUEBEC
800–463–5060 (Quebec only)

SASKATCHEWAN
306–359–4545

CONVENTIONAL TREATMENT

■ In the emergency care unit, charcoal may be instilled into your child's stomach in order to bind with the toxic substance and prevent it from being absorbed by the body.

■ Emergency personnel may perform *gastric lavage*, better known as stomach pumping. This procedure involves passing a tube through the nose and into the stomach to pump out the toxic substance.

■ Depending on the severity of the injury, your child may be admitted to a pediatric intensive care unit or a general pediatric unit for further treatment and/or observation.

■ An adolescent who has overdosed on a street drug may need to be hospitalized and treated depending on the drug and the amount ingested. If detoxification is needed, certain drugs may be given to ease symptoms of withdrawal. For instance, anti-anxiety medications such as Librium or valium may be used. Later on, methadone may be used to support an adolescent in maintaining abstinence from drugs. Individual, family, and group therapy, along with drug education and nutritional support are each important components of a recovery program. The following list of resources is for families dealing with drug or alcohol abuse.

Alateen and Al-Anon
  Family Groups
200 Park Avenue South
New York, NY 10003
212–254–7320

National Clearinghouse for
  Alcohol and Drug Information
PO Box 2345
Rockville, MD 20847–2345
301–468–2600

Alcoholics Anonymous
475 Riverside Drive
New York, NY 10115
212–870–3400

Families Anonymous
PO Box 528
Van Nuys, CA 90508
818–989–7841

GENERAL RECOMMENDATIONS

■ Once the crisis is over and your child has been medically evaluated, give her Bach Flower Rescue Remedy—three drops, three times a day, for one week. Rescue Remedy will help ease any fear, panic, anxiety, or tension.

■ Also following the crisis, it may be helpful to work with a professional health care practitioner to develop a program of nutritional therapies and natural support, including herbs and homeopathics, that will help detoxify the body and help it regain strength and health.

PREVENTION

■ The best way to prevent accidental poisoning is not to have poisonous products in your home at all. There are nontoxic alternatives to many poisonous commercial cleaning products. For example, mix equal parts of vinegar and water in a spray bottle to use as a glass cleaner. A handful of baking soda mixed with ½ cup of white vinegar can be used to help unclog a slow drain, replacing highly toxic drain cleaners. Baking soda makes as good a scouring powder as the commercial powders, which are loaded with bleach, detergents, and artificial dyes. *Nontoxic, Natural & Earthwise,* by Debra Lynn Dadd (J.P. Tarcher Inc., 1990) is a great reference to natural and homemade household products.

■ Dispose of toxic products responsibly—away from children and in a way that doesn't damage the earth. Call your state or local environmental administration, the Environmental Protection Agency, or your local health or sanitation department to find out how to dispose of hazardous materials. Ammonia cleaners, chlorine bleach, drain openers, furniture polish, and batteries (especially the "button batteries" used in watches and calculators) are examples of hazardous materials that should not be thrown away with your daily household garbage. And don't let the "empty" containers pile up in your basement or garage. Even tiny quantities of these toxins can do damage.

■ For suggestions on ways to childproof your home and guard against accidental poisonings, *see* HOME SAFETY in Part One.

Rash, Skin

See BITES AND STINGS, INSECT; FOOD ALLERGIES; POISON IVY, OAK, AND SUMAC.

Seizure

A seizure, or convulsion, is a sudden, uncontrollable contraction of a group of muscles. It may be mild or violent. When a child experiences a convulsion, all or part of his body may stiffen and jerk either with tiny, almost imperceptible movements, or with large, obvious movements.

Although a seizure usually lasts only a few minutes, seeing a child undergo one is a frightening experience for a parent. The child loses consciousness. His body may twitch or shake. His eyes may roll back and his teeth may clench. Breathing may be labored and heavy. The child may froth at the mouth, and he may wet himself.

Seizures can have a variety of causes, including high fever, a head injury, poisoning, shock, epilepsy, brain infection, or an allergic reaction. It may be an isolated occurrence or the result of a chronic disorder.

After a seizure has run its course, the child will sleep. Upon awakening, he will feel fatigued, disoriented, and dazed.

EMERGENCY TREATMENT FOR A SEIZURE

✚ Stay with your child. Talk reassuringly to him.

✚ Watch closely for changes in breathing and color. Be sure your child's airway stays open.

✚ Clear the area around your child to prevent injury, such as might occur if he knocks into a table or chair. Do not try to hold your child down. Restraining a thrashing child can cause additional injury.

✚ If vomiting occurs, turn your child's head to the side to prevent him from choking on inhaled vomit. If possible, keep his whole body turned on the side.

✚ *Do not* try to force anything into your child's mouth to hold down his tongue. You might cause him to choke, or you may suffer a bite yourself.

✚ Try to place a soft pillow or blanket under your child's head and loosen his clothing to prevent injury and ease discomfort.

✚ If the seizure lasts for less than ten minutes, allow your child to sleep afterwards, but keep watch and call your doctor.

✚ If the seizure lasts longer than ten minutes, or if your child is having difficulty breathing, is turning blue, or is hurting himself, call for emergency help.

✚ If your child has a seizure in combination with fever, vomiting, headache, irritability, lethargy, a stiff neck, or (in infants) a bulging fontanel (soft spot), call your doctor immediately. These can be signs of meningitis, a dangerous infection of the thin membranes that cover the brain and spinal cord.

✚ After a seizure, take your child to the doctor or hospital emergency room for an examination

GENERAL RECOMMENDATIONS

■ Once the seizure has passed and the crisis is over, give your child a dose of Bach Flower Rescue Remedy to help ease any fear, panic, anxiety, or tension.

■ Once your child has been evaluated and diagnosed, you may consider giving her supplemental magnesium for six weeks after a seizure. This helps to relax the nervous system.

Shock

Although many people use the word to describe an emotional reaction, in medical terms, shock is a physical state in which circulation is so severely compromised that blood cannot reach the body's tissues and organs. Without the essential nutrients and oxygen carried by the blood, the body becomes less and less able to perform its vital functions. This creates an emergency situation that requires immediate medical attention. If untreated, shock leads to complete circulatory collapse and death.

Shock can be caused by a variety of problems, including a severe allergic reaction, major blood loss, drug overdose, severe dehydration, serious infection, major emotional trauma (such as after a serious accident), or, in a person with diabetes, a sudden and dangerous rise in the amount of insulin in the body.

Signs and symptoms of shock include nausea, vomiting, weakness, cold and clammy skin, pale white or grayish skin color, dizziness, a cold sweat, increased breathing and heart rate, and restless or frightened behavior.

EMERGENCY TREATMENT
FOR SHOCK

✚ If an injured child appears to be in shock, call for emergency medical help immediately.

✚ While waiting for an ambulance to arrive, wrap the child in a warm blanket or extra clothes. Put a blanket between the child and the ground to help keep her body protected from the cool earth. If no blanket or extra clothing is available, use leaves, newspaper, or anything else on hand that can act as insulation.

✚ Keep the child on her back and raise her feet about a foot off the ground, so that they are at a level higher than her heart. If she has an injured arm or leg, raise it above the level of the heart as well. These measures decrease the workload of a heart that is already under stress.

✚ *If your child's breathing or pulse has stopped, turn to* CARDIOPUL-MONARY RESUSCITATION (CPR) *on page 33. Start CPR at once.*

✚ *If the child is bleeding, turn to* BLEEDING, SEVERE *on page 80. Take action immediately to stop the bleeding.*

✚ If the child is unknown to you, look for a Medic Alert necklace or bracelet that might explain the child's condition. For example, a child with diabetes may have a bracelet relating this information, which would guide medical personnel in their treatment.

✚ If the child vomits or begins bleeding from the mouth, turn her onto her side to prevent her from choking on inhaled fluid.

CONVENTIONAL TREATMENT

■ If shock is related to a large blood loss, your child will be given intravenous fluids to increase blood volume. Cardiopulmonary resuscitation (CPR), a blood transfusion, and/or a ventilator for breathing assistance may be required in severe situations.

■ If shock is caused by an allergic reaction, your child will be given epinephrine by injection to counteract the body's severe reaction to the allergen. Most often children respond to this treatment quickly and recover with little or no long-term treatment (*see* ANAPHYLACTIC REACTION).

GENERAL RECOMMENDATIONS

■ After emergency treatment has been administered and the crisis is over, give your child Bach Flower Rescue Remedy—three drops, three times a day, for one week. Rescue Remedy will help to ease any fear, panic, anxiety, or tension.

■ In addition to Rescue Remedy, give your child one dose of homeopathic *Aconite* 30c as soon as possible after the crisis to help easy any fright.

Shock, Electric

See ELECTRIC SHOCK.

Sprains and Strains

Both sprains and strains are injuries to the soft tissue—muscles, tendons, or ligaments. A strain is an injury to the muscle or tendon. A sprain, generally more serious than a strain, is an injury to the ligaments. Because ligaments connect bones to muscles, a sprained ligament can actually lead to more serious problems, such as dislocated joints. Both strains and sprains can be caused by overstretching, overuse, or specific traumatic events such as twisting an ankle on a soccer field or landing on a wrist while rollerblading.

Strains and sprains are graded according to the severity of the injury:

• A *grade-one* injury is a minor injury accompanied by mild pain and some swelling.

• A *grade-two* injury is characterized by moderate pain, bruising, and mild instability at the joint. The pain is likely to prevent the child from any physical activity. Touching or moving the injured area will cause increased pain.

- A *grade-three* injury is a complete or near-complete tear of a tendon or ligament. The injured area is very painful, swollen, and bruised. Because the supportive ligaments are torn, the child will not be able to use the affected area.

CONVENTIONAL TREATMENT

■ Immediately apply cold packs or immerse the area in cold water, especially if a sprain may be involved. Cold helps reduce swelling and inflammation. If possible, elevate the injured area. Apply cold for ten minutes every two hours.

■ If there is significant pain and swelling at the site of the injury, a trip to the doctor's office or the nearest emergency room is warranted. It is wise to have x-rays taken to evaluate the injury and make sure there are no broken bones. Being able to tell the doctor exactly what happened is helpful in diagnosis and treatment. Did the wrist turn in or out? Backwards or forwards? Was there any sound such as a snap or pop? Did you feel a tear or break?

■ To provide support, wrap the sprained area with an elastic bandage. Be careful not to wrap the area too tightly as this will interfere with circulation.

■ Try to have your child rest the area as much as possible. He should refrain from using or putting weight on the area until the pain and swelling are gone.

■ Surgery may be necessary if there is a complete tear of a ligament. Often this type of procedure can be done arthroscopically with local anesthesia.

■ Depending on the location and severity of the injury, a cast may be recommended. The current trend is to avoid rigid, permanent casts in favor of removable ones that can be worn during active times and taken off for bathing. Depending on the degree of injury, the cast may also be taken off for sleep. Follow the advice of your physician.

GENERAL RECOMMENDATIONS

■ Following a serious strain or sprain, physical therapy is important to rebuild strength and full range of motion to the joint. Have the therapist teach you the exercises, so you can help your child perform them at home regularly.

■ Custom orthotics, which are worn in the shoes to establish correct foot position, may be helpful for rehabilitation following a foot or ankle injury.

■ After proper treatment has been administered, homeopathic *Arnica* should be given as soon as possible to help reduce swelling. Give *Arnica* 30c, three times a day, for three days. After three days, give homeopathic *Ruta grav* 6c or 12x, three times a day, for three days. *Ruta grav* is useful after *Arnica* to help lessen the bruising, swelling, weakness, and pain to the injured area.

■ Apply homeopathic *Arnica* gel or Traumeel ointment to the bruise if the skin is not broken.

■ Bromelain, an enzyme extracted from pineapple stems, is a natural anti-inflammatory and can help reduce swelling. Give on an empty stomach.

■ Curcumin, the active ingredient in the herb turmeric, acts much like aspirin in helping to reduce swelling, pain, and inflammation. Concentrated curcumin is available in capsule form. For best results, take it with bromelain.

Sunburn

Sunburn is caused by exposure to radiation from the sun. It is usually a first-degree burn. In other words, it involves the epidermis, the outer (superficial) layer of the skin. If your child is sunburned, the exposed skin will be hot, red, and painful. If the skin blisters and swelling develops, a second-degree burn has occurred, and the dermis, the underlying layer of skin, has been affected (*see* BURNS).

The radiation that causes sunburn comes to the earth in the form of ultraviolet (UV) rays. There are two types of UV radiation: ultraviolet-A (UVA), which is present year round, and ultraviolet-B (UVB), which is present primarily in the summer months. While it was once believed that only UVB radiation presented the danger of damage from the sun, it is now known that UVA radiation is harmful also. As a result, experts recommend taking precautions against sun exposure no matter what the season.

A child's skin is tender and fragile. Without the protection of sun-screen, a hat, or clothing, it burns quickly. The sun's rays are further intensified when they are reflected by water or sand, and by suntan oils and lotions that do not contain sunscreen. Even if a child is wearing a T-shirt and sitting under a beach umbrella, reflected radiation can burn through the shirt.

A child's delicate skin should be sheltered from the sun. The long-term hazards of sun exposure have long been well known. More recent evidence suggests that skin cancer may be even more closely related to sunburn—even a single bad case, and especially a burn that occurs in childhood—than to total long-term sun exposure.

Just because your child doesn't seem to be getting burned as she plays outside, you cannot assume that she is unaffected by the sun's rays. A sunburn can develop and deepen even after your child is home and in bed. The pain of sunburn is most intense six to forty-eight hours after exposure to the sun. Skin that is lightly pinked when your child goes to bed may turn red, burning, and painful by the next morning. A severe sunburn can cause nausea, chills, and fever, as well as intense stinging.

WHEN TO CALL THE DOCTOR
ABOUT SUNBURN

Most cases of sunburn can be cared for at home, with natural remedies. Under certain circumstances, however, you should seek your doctor's advice:

• If your child's sunburned skin becomes blistered or swollen, call your health care provider. When blisters open, as with any open wound, there is an increased risk of infection.

• If a sunburned child develops secondary symptoms, such as chills, fever, or nausea, consult your physician. These may be signs of sun poisoning.

CONVENTIONAL TREATMENT

■ Painkillers such as ibuprofen and acetaminophen can be used to decrease the severity of sunburn pain if given soon after exposure but before a full-blown burn develops. If you give your child acetamino-phen, read the dosage instructions on the package carefully, as excessive amounts of this drug can cause liver damage. Ibuprofen is often best given with food to avoid possible stomach upset.

■ Cool showers, baths, or compresses are very soothing, and may prevent worsening of the burn, especially if used soon after sun exposure.

■ If your child suffers itching as a sunburn heals, an antihistamine such as Atarax, Benadryl, or Chlor-Trimeton may be recommended to counter the itching and swelling.

■ Anesthetic sprays that contain benzocaine are of value in some cases, especially if pain is severe. They can cause an allergic skin reaction and eczema in some children, however, and should not be used routinely on a child's sensitive skin.

■ For extremely severe sunburns, cortisone-like drugs such as prednisone may be prescribed to be taken orally or used in a topical spray. Although this can be dramatically effective when given early on, there are potentially serious side effects.

GENERAL RECOMMENDATIONS

■ If you suspect your child may be developing a sunburn, take her out of the sun right away.

■ To soothe and cool a sunburn quickly, apply aloe vera gel to the affected area.

■ After your child has been overexposed to the sun, have her soak in a cool bath. This will help to take the heat out of the burn, lessen the pain, and moisturize parched skin. Reapply aloe vera after the bath.

■ For an extra-soothing soak, treat your child's bath water with ½ cup of oatmeal (or Aveeno, a commercial product that is an oatmeal derivative). Wrap the oatmeal in a washcloth and let it soak in the tub. You can also *gently* rub the oatmeal-filled washcloth on your child's skin.

■ To soothe the worst areas of the burn, apply cool compresses where needed.

■ Dehydration often accompanies excessive exposure to the sun. Make sure your child gets sufficient fluids after spending time in the sun.

■ The homeopathic *Urtica urens* is effective in alleviating the stinging and burning pain of sunburn. Give *Urtica urens* 12x or 6c, every 15 minutes, up to four doses. You can also apply topical *Urtica urens* ointment or gel to the burn.

Tooth, Broken or Knocked Out

We often look at the structures of the mouth in a rather mechanical way—there are cavities, baby teeth, permanent teeth, perhaps braces. But if you think about the course of a child's development, you realize that for a newborn, his mouth is his primary means of communicating (through crying, cooing, and smiling) and of interacting with and learning about the world. His mouth brings relief of hunger as well as tranquil pleasure through suckling. Later, this versatile organ becomes a sensory probe for exploring our curious world—as we all know, babies and toddlers put *everything* in their mouths.

Fully one-third of the motor and sensory areas of the human brain are devoted to the mouth and oral structures. Disturbances here can therefore have far-reaching implications. Consequently, dental problems deserve serious attention. Among the most common tooth-related problems that affect children are the result of injuries.

Toddlers and older children may suffer mouth injuries that result in a tooth being fractured or knocked out. A toddler may sink his baby teeth into the corner of the coffee table or the linoleum floor during an attempt at a takeoff or landing. An older child can suffer a similar injury if he falls off his bicycle or is struck in the mouth by a softball. According to some estimates, injuries to the teeth account for as many as 50 percent of all childhood injuries.

Any child who suffers a tooth injury should be seen by a dentist, even if he seems to be fine afterwards. Complications such as an infection or abscess under the gum can develop and must be treated promptly. In addition, any tooth that has suffered trauma will have to be watched closely afterwards by your child's dentist. If your child has a baby tooth that was once pushed further into its socket, the permanent tooth that replaces it may emerge crooked or with some discoloration. Orthodontia and/or cosmetic dentistry may be necessary to treat the situation.

If your child suffers an injury that results in a fractured or knocked-out tooth, act quickly.

EMERGENCY TREATMENT
FOR A BROKEN OR KNOCKED-OUT TOOTH

✚ If your child has suffered a blow or injury to the mouth, wipe away any blood with a cool, clean, wet cloth and look at his teeth. If they are all present and properly aligned, check the *frenum* (the tissue that connects the lip to the gums) for lacerations.

✚ If a baby tooth is knocked out, don't worry about the tooth. However, if your child has a permanent tooth knocked out, and you find it within minutes, you should rinse it briefly to remove debris, but **do not** scrub it. Use one of the following (listed in order of preference) to rinse the tooth:

- A product called Save•A•Tooth, which is a nutrient-based solution designed specifically for this purpose. (Available in most pharmacies, Save•A•Tooth should be one of the items in your home health kit.)
- Physiologic saline solution (commercial eyewash).
- A cup (8 ounces) of water with ½ teaspoon of table salt dissolved in it.
- The child's own saliva.

✚ *Immediately* after rinsing the tooth, replace it in the tooth socket, checking its position with respect to adjacent teeth. Then call your dentist to explain the situation and arrange an emergency visit. If at all possible, it is better *not* to take the tooth to the dentist for reimplantation, but to replace it yourself and then seek your dentist's treatment. This will save precious time and prevent clotting from taking place in the socket. Also, immediately after an injury, the shock will cause your child's face to feel somewhat numb. If the tooth is reimplanted after this numbness (as well as the distraction of the event) has passed, this process will be needlessly difficult for your child.

✚ If all of your child's teeth are present but one appears to have been displaced deeper into the socket, clasp the bone and palate above the tooth firmly between your thumb and finger. Firmly but gently squeeze/massage with a downward motion to encourage the tooth to return to a normal position. Call your dentist to explain the situation and arrange an emergency visit.

✚ If your child has fractured a tooth, call your dentist. Tooth fractures vary in severity, depending on the amount of the inner tooth that has been exposed, and the severity is what determines the appropriate treatment. A chip or a very shallow fracture, for example, may require only cosmetic treatment—the fracture smoothed out to eliminate rough or sharp edges. In such a case, the newly exposed area of tooth will calcify in time and become less sensitive as long as it is kept clean, brushed with a mineralizing toothpaste, and kept from contact with decalcifying foods such as carbonated sodas and apples. If the fracture is somewhat deeper, your dentist may recommend restoring it by means of bonding techniques.

✚ A deeply fractured tooth requires immediate treatment to prevent infection and other complications. If your child suffers a deep tooth fracture, if possible, rinse the broken part quickly and hold it in place until it can be treated. Or place clean plastic wrap over the bleeding area and have your child secure it by biting steadily on a piece of folded gauze. This will seal off and protect the injured area until you can get to your dentist's office. If possible, save the broken piece of the tooth; it may be possible for your dentist to reattach it. Call your dentist to arrange an emergency visit.

✚ If a fracture is particularly severe, root canal therapy may be advised. A root canal is a procedure in which the nerve is removed and replaced with a sterile material such as a heavy wax or paste. Root canals are a source of controversy in dentistry, as they expose the immune system to mixtures of different metals and other foreign substances, some of which may have toxic or immune-compromising effects. Unfortunately, if a tooth is injured or decayed badly enough, there are, as yet, few alternatives except extraction. There is some research that suggests root canals may be better tolerated if they are performed before a tooth becomes seriously degenerated. Before agreeing to have root canal therapy performed on your child's tooth, it is a good idea to discuss with your dentist all of the available treatment options and the pros and cons of each for your individual child's situation.

GENERAL RECOMMENDATIONS

■ After proper emergency treatment has been administered, give your child Bach Flower Rescue Remedy—three drops, three times a day, for a week. Rescue Remedy will help ease any fear, panic, anxiety, or tension.

■ In addition to Rescue Remedy, give your child one dose of homeopathic *Arnica* 30c or *Aconite* 30c to help ease any fright.

■ To help alleviate any nerve pain, give your child homeopathic *Hypericum* 30c, three times a day, for three days.

PREVENTION

■ There are some injuries a parent cannot prevent. You can, however, reduce the possibility that your child will suffer a mouth injury by taking measures to childproof your house. *See* HOME SAFETY in Part One.

■ Be prepared. Keep Save•A•Tooth solution on hand in case your child knocks out or fractures a tooth. It is available in many drugstores or it can be ordered from the manufacturer, Biological Rescue Products, by calling 800–882–0505. It is a good idea to order two—one for home and one for the car. This nutrient-based product is simple to use, and research has shown that it can keep a tooth alive for hours if it cannot be reimplanted immediately (without protection, a knocked-out tooth will often die in about fifteen minutes). This reduces the possibility that a tooth will be permanently lost, causing your child stress and embarrassment and creating the need for years of expensive dental procedures and exposure to metal bridgework.

■ Teach your child to be appropriately cautious and thoughtful in all of his activities. Insist on proper headgear for activities like bicycling, skiing, and contact sports such as football or hockey. When riding in a car, always wear your seat belt and make sure your child does the same. A baby should always ride in an approved child restraint seat.

■ Proper oral hygiene and regular visits to the dentist are important. A decaying tooth is much more likely to chip or fracture than a healthy tooth. A good program of oral care should begin as soon as your baby is born—even before any teeth erupt.

Unconsciousness

See also FAINTING.

A child who has lost consciousness may be in serious difficulty. An unconscious state signals a lack of adequate oxygen supply to the brain. Causes may include shock and breathing problems, such as choking and near-suffocation. A loss of consciousness can also be caused by the ingestion of drugs or poisons. Other possible causes are brain injury, seizures, stroke, brain tumor, and infection.

Fainting is a term used to describe a less serious episode in which consciousness is lost. This is caused by a temporary disruption of blood flow to the brain, which may be brought on by hunger or pain, or even overwhelming emotional circumstances. Fainting is usually momentary, and a child who has fainted will revive readily, without disorientation upon awakening, although she may feel fatigued.

If unconsciousness lasts for more than a few minutes, however, there may be other problems, such as internal or external bleeding, which can lead to shock. If your child loses consciousness, try to remain calm and act quickly.

EMERGENCY TREATMENT
FOR UNCONSCIOUSNESS

✚ Call the child's name. Try to provoke a response by sharply patting your child's face. Shake her gently. If she does not respond immediately, use smelling salts or an open bottle of perfume to help revive her.

✚ If your child is limp and does not respond, call for emergency help immediately. It is best to have someone else call, so that your child is not left alone. If you must make the call yourself, do not leave your child unattended for more than thirty seconds.

✚ Quickly assess the situation. If you suspect that your child may have suffered a neck or back injury, such as might occur in a fall, **do not** move or jostle her. Rely on emergency medical personnel to know how to stabilize your child so that transport to the hospital will be safe.

✚ If you do not suspect a neck or back injury, turn your child onto her back. Roll her whole body as a unit to prevent further injury.

✚ Check for breathing. Put your cheek close to your child's mouth to feel for a breath. Watch her chest to see if it is rising and falling in normal breathing.

✚ *If your child's breathing or pulse has stopped, turn to* CARDIOPULMONARY RESUSCITATION (CPR) *on page 33. Start CPR at once.*

✚ Once your child's pulse and breathing have been restored and the immediate crisis is over, check and treat your child for bleeding, broken bones, concussion, or any other injury or problem she might have (*see* BLEEDING, INTERNAL; BLEEDING, SEVERE; BONES, BROKEN; CONCUSSION).

✚ After any episode during which your child loses consciousness, it is wise to call your physician or take your child to the emergency room of the nearest hospital. Even if your child seems to be fine after such an ordeal, she should be seen by a doctor. It is important to seek the advice of a qualified medical professional.

GENERAL RECOMMENDATIONS

■ Once the emergency is over and your child has been medically evaluated, give her Bach Flower Rescue Remedy—three drops, three times a day, for one week. Rescue Remedy will help ease any fear, panic, anxiety, or tension.

About the Authors

Janet Zand, Lac, OMD, has been a practitioner of natural medicine for the past nineteen years. She uses homeopathy, herbal medicine, acupuncture, nutritional medicine, exercise, and lifestyle modification to create an integrated approach to optimum health. Dr. Zand is also a frequent lecturer and a widely quoted authority on natural medicine. In addition, she has formulated many popular herbal and nutritional medicines. She resides in Malibu, California.

Rachel Walton, RN, MSN, is a pediatric nurse with a master's degree in child health nursing from the Massachusetts General Hospital Institute of Health Professions. She has worked with children and families facing chronic and terminal illness, in general pediatrics, and in postpartum home care. She teaches classes to new mothers on using natural medicine to take care of their babies and young children. She lives in Boulder, Colorado.

Bob Rountree, MD, received his medical degree from the University of North Carolina School of Medicine and completed a three-year residency in family and community medicine at the Milton S. Hershey Medical Center in Hershey, Pennsylvania, after which he was certified by the American Board of Family Practice. He has done extensive postgraduate study in nutritional and herbal pharmacology, and has received certification as a master practitioner of neuro-linguistic programming. Dr. Rountree has been practicing medicine in Boulder, Colorado, since 1983, providing a unique combination of traditional family medicine, nutrition, herbology, and mind-body therapy.

Index

A

Index

Atarax, 169
Aveeno, 169
Azmacort, 68

B

B vitamins, 61. *See also* Vitamin B$_{12}$.
Bach Flower Rescue Remedy, 16, 60, 62, 64, 97, 99, 109, 111, 118, 124, 135, 160, 163, 165, 172, 175
Bacitracin, 70, 91, 101, 146
Back, injured, immobilizing, 44–45. *See also* Bones, broken.
Back injury. *See* Bones, broken.
Bandage, pressure, applying, 46–48
Barley malt, 16, 105
Beclovent, 68
Bee stings, 74–75. *See also* Bites and stings, insect.
Belladonna, homeopathic, 16, 123
Benadryl, 64, 125, 133, 148, 169
    proper dosage for, 18
Benzocaine, 168
Betadine, 70, 91, 101
Bifidus, 62, 128, 140
Bioflavonoids, 88, 92
Bites, animal and human, 69–71
    conventional treatment for, 70
    emergency treatment for, 69–70
    general recommendations for, 71

    See also Bites, snake; Bites and stings, insect.
Bites, snake, 71–73
    conventional treatment for, 72
    emergency treatment for, 71–72
    general recommendations for, 72–73
    prevention of, 73
Bites and stings, insect, 73–78
    emergency treatment for, 74–76
    general recommendations for, 76–77
    prevention of, 77–78
Black eye. *See* Eye injuries.
Bleeding, internal, 78–80
    conventional treatment for, 79
    emergency treatment for, 79
    general recommendations for, 80
    See also Bleeding, severe.
Bleeding, nose. *See* Nosebleed.
Bleeding, severe, 46–48, 80–84
    conventional treatment for, 83–84
    emergency treatment for, 81–83
    general recommendations for, 84
    See also Bleeding, internal; Cuts and scrapes; Nosebleed.
Bones, broken, 84–86
    conventional treatment for, 85–86
    emergency treatment for, 85

I

K

L